The Low Gi Guide

to the Metabolic Syndrome and Your Heart

Dr Jennie Brand-Miller
the authority on low GI eating
Kaye Foster-Powell, Dr Anthony Leeds

Copyright © 2003, 1998 Jennie Brand-Miller, Kaye Foster-Powell and Anthony Leeds

First published by Hodder Headline Australia
This edition first published in Great Britain in 2005 by
Hodder and Stoughton
A division of Hodder Headline

This United Kingdom edition is published by arrangement with
Hodder Headline Australia Pty Limited

The right of Jennie Brand-Miller, Kaye Foster-Powell and
Anthony Leeds to be identified as the Authors of the Work has
been asserted by them in accordance with the Copyright,
Designs and Patents Act 1988

A Mobius Book

1 3 5 7 9 10 8 6 4 2

A CIP catalogue record for this title is available from the British Library.

ISBN 0340 896027

Typeset by Egan-Reid Ltd, Auckland

Printed and bound by Clays Ltd, St Ives plc

Hodder Headline's policy is to use papers that are natural, renewable and recyclable products and made from wood grown in sustainable forests. The logging and manufacturing processes are expected to conform to the environmental regulations of the country of origin.

Hodder and Stoughton Ltd
A division of Hodder Headline
338 Euston Road
London NW1 3BH

CONTENTS

FOREWORD

There have been many popular diets that, although widely publicised, have had little scientific backing. In contrast, the evidence for a diet based on foods with a low glycaemic index is good.

Some of today's major killers confronted in medical practice are the result of obesity. Many overweight patients are suffering from the metabolic syndrome because of obesity. Too many discover too late that the metabolic syndrome can lead to diabetes, heart disease, high blood pressure, polycystic ovaries and a host of other problems. The metabolic syndrome is destined to become increasingly well known, even notorious, once it is more widely recognised and better understood. Part of the answer to the metabolic syndrome is an aware-ness of the glycaemic index, what it means and the advantages that will follow if note is taken of it. The way to discover more about the syndrome is to read *The Low GI Guide to the Metabolic Syndrome and Your Heart*, a well written and explicit but easily understood book by Dr Anthony Leeds, Senior Lecturer at King's College London and his Sydney colleagues, Professor Jennie Brand-Miller, Professor of Human Nutrition at the University of Sydney and Kaye Foster-Powell, an accredited practising dietitian.

Dr Tom Stuttaford
Medical Correspondent, *The Times*

INTRODUCTION

Did you know that heart disease is the single biggest killer in the UK? Every minute, every day, someone in the UK suffers a cardiovascular event. So what causes this deadly disease? Often it is a result of atherosclerosis or 'hardening of the arteries'. We now know it's not just a 'plumbing' problem, but one in which inflammation plays a key role.

Heart disease, however, seldom occurs as an isolated condition. One in two Britons over 25 years of age has at least two features of the 'silent' disease: the metabolic syndrome (sometimes called the insulin resistance syndrome or Syndrome X). The metabolic syndrome is a collection of metabolic abnormalities—like a 'pot belly', high blood pressure, high blood glucose, low levels of 'good' cholesterol—that increase your risk of atherosclerosis and heart attack.

While most people these days are aware of the importance of cutting back on fat to minimise their risk of heart disease, very few people are aware that the type of carbohydrate they eat can also help prevent heart disease and improve the metabolic syndrome.

Research on the glycaemic index of foods, what we have called the GI, shows that the type of carbohydrate we eat may have as much influence on our risk of heart disease as the type of fat we eat.

As we explain in our bestselling book, *The New Glucose Revolution*, the glycaemic index:

- is a scientifically proven measure of the effect carbohydrates have on blood glucose levels;
- helps you choose the right amount and type of carbohydrate for your health and wellbeing;
- provides an easy and effective way to eat a healthy diet and control fluctuations in blood glucose.

It's vital that people learn about the GI so they base their food choices on sound scientific evidence.

What is the GI?

The glycaemic index (GI) is a physiologically based measure of carbohydrate quality—a comparison of carbohydrates (gram for gram) based on their immediate effect on blood glucose levels.

- Carbohydrates that break down quickly during digestion have **high GI** values. Their blood glucose response is fast and high.
- Carbohydrates that break down slowly, releasing glucose gradually into the blood stream, have a **low GI**.

The rate of carbohydrate digestion has important implications for everybody. For more detailed information about the glycaemic index and its many benefits you should consult *The New Glucose Revolution* or *The Low GI Life Plan*. And for those looking to lose weight, please refer to the 12-week action plan featured in *The Low GI Diet*. These books published by Hodder Mobius are available from all good bookshops.

WHAT THIS BOOK CAN DO FOR YOU

Understanding the GI has made an enormous difference to the diet and lifestyle of many people. Recent studies show that diets rich in slowly digested carbohydrates with a low glycaemic index:

- reduce blood cholesterol levels
- reduce the 'bad' LDL cholesterol
- increase the 'good' HDL cholesterol
- reduce CRP (a measure of chronic, low-grade inflammation)
- increase the body's sensitivity to insulin
- improve blood flow
- reduce hunger
- help weight control

In practical terms this means that:

- your intake of bread, potatoes, rice and pasta can influence your risk of heart disease;
- a diet rich in quickly digested carbohydrates may increase your risk of a heart attack; and
- eating more fruit, wholegrains, dried peas and lentils, and beans and low fat dairy foods can reduce your risk of heart disease.

In this book we will show you how vitally important an understanding of the GI is for your heart health and how easy it is to make the change to a low GI diet. We will:

- explain how the GI is measured;
- outline the beneficial aspects of the GI for heart health;
- show you how to include more of the right sort of carbohydrate in your diet;
- give practical hints to help you make the GI work for you throughout the day;
- provide a week of low GI menus with nutritional analysis; and
- list the GI of over 350 foods for easy reference.

UNDERSTANDING THE GLYCAEMIC INDEX

The glycaemic index (GI) concept was first developed in 1981 by Dr David Jenkins, a professor of nutrition at the University of Toronto, Canada, to help determine which carbohydrates were best for people with diabetes. At that time, the diet for people with diabetes was based on a system of carbohydrate exchanges, which assumed that all starchy foods produced the same effect on blood glucose levels, even though earlier studies had already proven this was not correct. Jenkins was one of the first people to question this assumption and investigate how real foods behave in the bodies of real people.

Since then, scientists, including the authors of this book, have tested the effect of different foods on blood glucose levels and other biochemical factors. Clinical studies in the United Kingdom, France, Italy, Australia and Canada all have proven the value of the glycaemic index.

The GI of foods is simply a ranking of carbohydrates in foods according to their immediate impact on blood glucose levels. To make a fair comparison, all foods are compared with a reference food such as pure glucose and are tested in equivalent carbohydrate amounts.

Today we know the GI of hundreds of different food items that have been tested following the standardised method. We have included many of these values in the tables at the back of this book, but for more detailed information you should consult *The New Glucose Revolution* or *The Low GI Shopper's Guide to GI Values*.

The key is the rate of digestion

Foods containing carbohydrates that break down quickly during digestion have the highest GI value. The blood glucose response is fast and high (in other words, the glucose in the bloodstream increases rapidly). Conversely, foods that contain carbohydrates which break down slowly, releasing glucose gradually into the bloodstream, have low GI values.

For most people, the foods with a low GI have advantages over those with high GI values. This is especially true for those people trying to prevent the metabolic syndrome and atherosclerosis.

The higher the GI, the higher the blood glucose levels after consumption of the food. Instant white rice (GI of 87) and baked potatoes (GI of 85) have very high GIs, meaning their effect on blood glucose levels is almost as high as that of an equal amount of pure glucose (yes, you read it correctly).

Low GI = 55 or less
Moderate/Medium GI = 56 to 69
High GI = 70 or more

Figure 1 shows the blood glucose response to potatoes compared with pure glucose. Foods with a low GI (like lentils at 29) show a flatter blood glucose response when eaten, as shown in Figure 2. The peak blood glucose level is lower and the return to baseline levels is slower than with a high GI food.

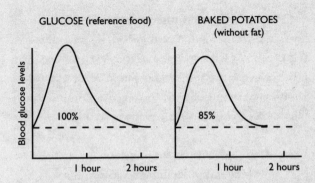

Figure 1. The effect of pure glucose (50 g) and baked potatoes without fat (50 g carbohydrate portion) on blood glucose levels.

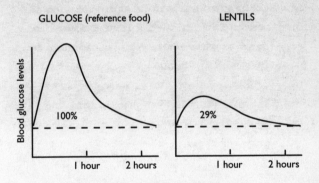

Figure 2. The effect of pure glucose (50 g) and lentils (50 g carbohydrate portion) on blood glucose levels.

How we measure the GI

Pure glucose produces the greatest rise in blood glucose levels. Most foods have less effect when fed in equal carbohydrate quantities. The GI of pure glucose is set at 100 and every other food is ranked on a scale from 1 to 100 according to its actual effect on blood glucose levels.

1. An amount of food containing a standard amount of carbohydrate (usually 25 or 50 grams) is given to a volunteer to eat. For example, to test boiled spaghetti, the volunteer will be given 200 grams of spaghetti which supplies 50 grams of carbohydrate (determined from food composition tables).

2. Over the next two hours (or three hours if the volunteer has diabetes), we take a sample of their blood every 15 minutes during the first hour and thereafter every 30 minutes. The blood glucose level of these blood samples is measured in the laboratory and recorded.

3. The blood glucose level is plotted on a graph and the area under the curve is calculated using a computer programme (Figure 3).

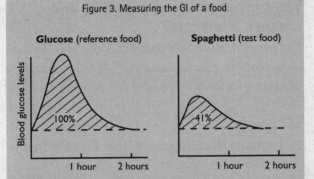

Figure 3. Measuring the GI of a food

The test food and the reference food must contain the same amount of carbohydrate. The usual dose is 50 grams but sometimes 25 grams is used when the portion size would be otherwise too large. Even smaller doses such as 15 grams have been used. The GI result is much the same whatever the dose because the GI is simply a relative measure of carbohydrate quality.

4. The volunteer's response to spaghetti (or whatever food is being tested) is compared with his or her blood glucose response to 50 grams of pure glucose (the reference food).

5. The reference food is tested on two or three separate occasions and an average value is calculated. This is done to reduce the effect of day-to-day variation in blood glucose responses.

6. The average GI found in 8–10 people is the GI of that food.

What gives one food a high GI and another a low one?

The physical state of the starch in the food is the most important factor influencing the GI. That's why food processing has such a profound effect on the GI.

Factors that influence the GI of a food

Factor	Mechanism	Examples of food where the effect is seen
Starch gelatinisation	The less gelatinised (swollen) the starch, the slower the rate of digestion.	Spaghetti, porridge, biscuits have less gelatinised starch.
Physical entrapment	The fibrous coat around beans and seeds and plant cell walls acts as a physical barrier, slowing down access of enzymes to the starch inside.	Pumpernickel and grainy bread, legumes and barley.
High amylose to amylopectin ratio*	The more amylose a food contains, the less easily the starch is gelatinised and the slower its rate of digestion.	Basmati rice contains more amylose than other types of rice.
Particle size	The smaller the particle size, the easier it is for water and enzymes to penetrate (the surface area is relatively higher).	Finely milled flours have high GIs. Stone-ground flours have larger particles and lower GIs.

Factors that influence the GI of a food *(cont.)*

Factor	Mechanism	Examples of food where the effect is seen
Viscosity of fibre	Viscous, soluble fibres increase the viscosity of the intestinal contents and this slows down the interaction between the starch and the enzymes. Finely milled wholemeal wheat and rye flours have fast rates of digestion and absorption because the fibre is not viscous.	Rolled oats, beans and lentils, apples.
Sugar	The digestion of sugar produces only half as many glucose molecules as the same amount of starch (the other half is fructose). The presence of sugar also restricts gelatinisation of the starch by binding water and reducing the amount of 'available' water.	Some biscuits, some breakfast cereals that are high in sugar have relatively low GI values.
Acidity	Acids in foods slow down stomach emptying, thereby slowing the rate at which the starch can be digested.	Vinegar, lemon juice, lime juice, salad dressings, pickled vegetables, sourdough bread.
Fat	Fat slows down the rate of stomach emptying, thereby slowing the digestion of the starch.	Potato crisps have a lower GI than boiled potatoes.

* Amylose and amylopectin are two different types of starch. Both are found in foods, but the ratio varies.

WHAT IS HEART DISEASE?

As we mentioned earlier most heart disease is caused by atherosclerosis of the arteries, sometimes referred to as 'hardening of the arteries'. Generally, people develop atherosclerosis gradually during their lifetime and live much of their life blissfully unaware of it. If it develops fairly slowly it may not cause any problems, even into great old age, but if its development is accelerated by one or more of many processes (such as high cholesterol or high glucose levels) the condition may cause trouble much earlier in life.

Atherosclerosis

Atherosclerosis results in reduced blood flow through the affected arteries. In the heart this can mean that the heart muscle gets insufficient oxygen to provide the power for pumping blood and it changes in such a way that pain is experienced (central chest pain or angina pectoris). Elsewhere in the body, atherosclerosis has a similar blood flow reducing effect: in the legs it can cause muscle pains on exercise; in the brain it can cause a variety of problems from 'funny turns' to strokes.

An even more serious consequence of atherosclerosis occurs when a blood clot forms over the surface of a patch of atherosclerosis on an artery. This process of thrombosis can result in a complete blockage of the artery, with consequences ranging from sudden death to a small heart attack from which the patient generally recovers quickly.

The process of thrombosis can occur elsewhere in the arterial system with outcomes determined by the extent of the thrombosis. The probability of developing thrombosis is determined by the 'tendency' of the blood to clot versus the natural ability of the blood to break down clots (fibrinolysis). These two counteracting 'tendencies' are influenced by a number of factors, including the level of glucose in the blood.

> Knowing your blood glucose level is just as important as knowing your cholesterol level.

People who have gradually developed atherosclerosis of the arteries to the heart (the coronary arteries) may slowly develop reduced heart function. For a while the heart may be able to compensate for the problem, so there are no symptoms, but eventually it begins to fail. Shortness of breath may occur, initially on exercise, and sometimes there may be some swelling of the ankles. Atherosclerosis can also lead to abnormal heart beat (palpitations).

Modern medicine has many effective drug treatments for heart failure so this consequence of atherosclerosis does not have quite the same serious implications as it did in the past.

Why do people get heart disease?

For most people atherosclerotic heart disease develops early in life when the many factors that cause it have a strong influence. Over many decades doctors and scientists have identified the processes which cause heart disease in fine detail and now most of the factors are well known.

Theoretically, atherosclerotic heart disease might be largely prevented if everyone's risks were assessed in youth and then if all the right things were done throughout the rest of their lives. In practice, there has been limited development of the ways to screen people for risk early in life, and the resources needed to achieve prevention are just not available.

A great deal is already being done, however, to identify risk factors (i.e. 'red flags') in healthy people and those with established heart disease. A high cholesterol level is a well-established risk factor, as is a low level of HDL—the 'good' cholesterol.

More recently, high glucose levels after eating have been shown to be an important, but under-recognised predictor of both cardiovascular disease and death from any cause. High levels of glucose in the blood, even transient increases such as after a meal, have many undesirable effects, stemming from the fact that glucose increases the production of 'free radicals'. Free radicals are highly reactive, charged molecules that inflict harm on everything close by. They damage proteins, fats and cellular structures. In particular, they cause inflammation of the cells lining blood vessels. We now recognise that atherosclerosis is an inflammatory disease.

The good news is that those of us who take the necessary action will reduce our risk.

We discuss the risk factors for heart disease further on pages 28–34.

> High glucose levels after eating have been shown to be an important predictor of cardiovascular disease. A low GI diet helps reduce post-meal blood glucose levels.

HOW CAN THE GI HELP?

The type of carbohydrate we eat determines the body's blood glucose response and also determines the levels of insulin in our blood for many hours after eating. High insulin levels caused by eating foods with a high GI are undesirable. In the long term, they promote high blood fat, high blood glucose, high blood pressure and increase the risk of heart attack.

Because of this, the GI of the diet is significant in the long-term prevention of heart disease and may be equally important in the diets of people who already have heart disease.

Firstly, a low GI diet has benefits for weight control, helping to satisfy appetite and preventing overeating and excessive body weight.

Secondly, it helps reduce post-meal blood glucose levels in both normal and diabetic individuals. This improves the elasticity of the walls of the arteries, making dilation easier and improving blood flow.

Thirdly, blood fats and clotting factors can be improved by low GI diets.

Low GI diets also reduce total blood cholesterol and low-density (LDL) cholesterol in people with undesirably high levels. Lower levels of total cholesterol and LDL cholesterol are associated with a lower risk of heart disease.

Specifically, population studies have shown that HDL cholesterol levels are correlated with the GI and glycaemic load of the diet. Those of us who self-select the lowest GI diets have the highest and best levels of HDL—the good cholesterol.

HDL cholesterol is a sign of cholesterol being taken away from arteries, so the higher the levels the better. Large scale surveys have shown that high HDL cholesterol is the best predictor of a lower risk of heart disease. One of the key features of the metabolic syndrome is a low HDL level.

Furthermore, research studies in people with diabetes have shown that low GI diets reduce triglycerides in the blood, a factor strongly linked to the metabolic syndrome. Lastly, low GI diets have been shown to improve insulin sensitivity in people at high risk of heart disease, thereby helping to reduce the rise in blood glucose and insulin levels after normal meals.

By working on several fronts at one time, low GI diets have a distinct advantage over other types of diets or drugs that target only one risk factor at a time.

One study in particular has provided the best evidence in support of the role of the GI in heart disease. The study was conducted by Harvard University and is commonly referred to as 'the Nurses Study'. The Nurses Study is an ongoing, long-term study of over 100 000 nurses who provide their personal health and diet information to researchers at Harvard School of Public Health every few years. In this way, diet can be linked with the future development of different diseases. It found that those who ate more high GI foods had nearly twice the risk of having a heart attack over a ten-year period of follow-up, compared to those eating low GI diets. This association was independent of dietary fibre and other known risk factors, such as age and body mass index. In other words, even if fibre intake was high, there was still an adverse effect of high GI diets on risk. Importantly, neither sugar nor total carbohydrate intake showed any association with risk of heart attack. Thus there was no evidence that lower carbohydrate or sugar intake was helpful.

One of the most important findings of the Nurses Study was that the increased risk associated with high GI diets was largely seen in those with a body mass index (BMI) over 23. (To calculate your body mass divide your weight in kilograms by the square of your height in metres.) There was no increased risk in those under 23. But the fact remains that the great majority of adults have a BMI greater than 23; indeed a BMI of 23–25 is considered normal weight. The implication therefore is that the insulin resistance that comes with increasing weight is an integral part of the disease process. So, if you are very lean and insulin sensitive, high GI diets won't make you more prone to heart attack. This might explain why traditional-living Asian populations, such as the Chinese, who eat high GI rice as a staple food, do not show increased risk of heart disease. Their low BMI and their high level of physical activity conspire to keep them insulin sensitive and extremely carbohydrate tolerant.

The GI may reduce the risk of heart disease by increasing the 'good' cholesterol and reducing the level of triglycerides (fats) in the blood.

Treating the metabolic syndrome and heart disease

When the metabolic syndrome or actual signs of heart disease are detected two types of treatment are given. Firstly, the effects of the disease are treated (e.g. medical treatment with drugs and surgical treatment to bypass blocked arteries) and, secondly, the risk factors are treated to slow down further progression of the disease.

Treatment of risk factors after the disease has already developed is 'secondary prevention'. In people who have not yet developed the disease (e.g. those with insulin resistance), treatment of risk factors is 'primary prevention'.

Obviously it would be better to give primary preventive treatment in all cases, but the GI has application in both cases.

Preventing heart disease

More and more people now get regular checks of their blood pressure, and tests to check for diabetes. Increasingly, blood cholesterol tests are done to check this risk factor too. If your medical practitioner is on the ball, he or she will also do a blood glucose test.

All health professionals give lifestyle advice on stopping smoking, the benefits of exercise and the nature of a good diet. When specific risk factors are discovered, diet and lifestyle advice is given, but sometimes may not be followed for long.

It is especially difficult to follow advice if the effect of not following it is likely not to matter for ten or more years, and if the changes needed are not attractive. The changes must be wanted by the individual who will be helped by encouragement from friends and relatives, and the changes must ideally be positive changes—'I want to do this', not 'They've told me to do this.'

TEST YOUR HEART KNOWLEDGE

Try this quick quiz on diet and heart disease to test your knowledge. Answer true or false to the following:

1. All vegetable oils are low in saturated fat.
2. Butter contains more fat than margarine.
3. Britons eat more fat now than 10 years ago.
4. Eggs should be avoided on a low fat, cholesterol-lowering diet.
5. Moderate consumption of alcohol increases your risk of heart attack.
6. Olive oil has the lowest fat content of any oil.
7. A cup of milk contains less fat than two squares of chocolate.
8. Nuts will raise cholesterol levels.
9. Potatoes and pasta are fattening foods.
10. Cod liver oil will lower cholesterol levels.

The answer to each of the preceding questions is false. Here's an explanation why …

1. Contrary to popular belief, not all vegetable oils are low in saturated fat. Two primary exceptions are coconut oil and palm or palm kernel oil. Both these oils (which may appear on a food label simply as vegetable oil) are highly saturated. Palm oil is used widely in commercial cakes, biscuits, pastries and fried foods.

2. Butter and margarine contain similar levels of fat (around 85–90 per cent). There is a difference in the types of fats which predominate, however, butter being about 60 per cent saturated fat and unsaturated margarines being less than 30 per cent saturated fat.

3. Britons are eating less fat now than 10 years ago. In 1988, we ate 35 per cent of our energy in the form of fat. Now we are down to 32 per cent but we still have a way to go to achieve 30 per cent. Plus, these are average figures, so many of us are still eating far too much fat.

4. Eggs are a source of cholesterol but dietary cholesterol tends to raise blood cholesterol levels only when the background diet is high in fat. One egg contains only about 5 grams of fat, of which only 2 grams is saturated.

5. Moderate amounts of alcohol (e.g. 2 standard drinks per day) appear to reduce the risk of heart attack. Amounts in excess are harmful to health.

6. There is no such thing as low fat oil. Oil is fat in a liquid form, its fat content being 100 per cent. Olive oil is a suitable choice of oils containing only 15 per cent saturated fats. Mediterranean populations, whose major source of fat is olive oil, have low levels of heart disease.

7. Half a pint (250 ml) of full cream milk contains 9.7 grams of fat. Compare this to about four grams contained in two small squares of chocolate!

8. Nuts have been found to be protective against heart disease. While most nuts are high in fat, much of the fat they contain is of the 'good' monounsaturated and polyunsaturated types.

9. This myth has been around for years. Potatoes and pasta are high carbohydrate foods which means they are a good source of energy for the body. They are rarely stored as body fat.

10. Cod liver oil has not been found to lower cholesterol levels. It is extremely rich in vitamins A and D and should not be taken in large doses because of the danger of vitamin A toxicity.

HEART DISEASE RISK FACTORS

Your chance of developing heart disease is increased if you smoke tobacco, have high blood pressure, have diabetes or 'pre-diabetes' (high glucose levels but not yet as high as in diabetes), have high blood cholesterol (which may be due to eating too much saturated fat in your diet), are overweight or obese and/or sedentary.

Low saturated fat and low GI diets help prevent heart disease.

Smoking

Smoking tobacco is now clearly established as a cause of atherosclerosis. Few authorities dispute the evidence. There are, however, some interesting dietary aspects. Did you know that:

- smokers tend to eat less fruit and vegetables compared to non-smokers (and thus eat less of the protective anti-oxidant plant compounds); and
- smokers tend to eat more fat and more salt than non-smokers?

These characteristics of the smoker's diet may be caused by a desire to seek strong food flavours as a consequence of the taste-blunting effect of smoking. While these dietary differences may make the smoker at greater risk of heart disease there is only one piece of advice for anyone who smokes:

Please stop smoking!

High blood pressure

High blood pressure (hypertension) is very damaging because it demands that your heart work harder and it damages your arteries. Remember, an artery is not a rigid pipe, it is a muscular tube, which when healthy can change its size to control the flow of blood.

High blood pressure causes changes in the walls of arteries which makes atherosclerosis more likely to develop. Blood clots can then form and the weakened blood vessels can easily thrombose or rupture and bleed. In Britain, approximately 1 in 2 people aged 65 years and over is hypertensive.

Treatments for blood pressure have become more effective over the last thirty years, but it is only now becoming clear which types of treatment for blood pressure are also effective at reducing heart disease risk.

Normal range for blood pressure:

Less than 140/90 mm Hg

Diabetes and 'pre-diabetes'

Diabetes is, in itself, a further risk factor for heart disease. Diabetes is caused by a lack of insulin—either the body does not produce enough, or the body 'demands' more than normal (because it has become insensitive to insulin). Diabetes and pre-diabetes (impaired glucose tolerance) cause inflammation and hardening of the arteries. When glucose levels are raised, even temporarily (such as after eating), oxidising reactions are accelerated and the level of anti-oxidants such as vitamin E and C decline. In particular, the blood fats are oxidised, making them more damaging to artery walls. The walls become inflamed, thicken and gradually lose their elasticity. The constriction of the arteries results in increased blood pressure. If that's not bad enough, high insulin levels increase the tendency for blood clots to form. The resulting increased risk of heart attack is a major reason why we put so much effort into helping people with diabetes achieve normal control of blood glucose and also why all people with diabetes should be checked for the other risk factors of heart disease. But you don't need to have diabetes to be at risk—even moderately raised blood glucose levels hours after a meal have been associated with increased risk of heart disease in normal 'healthy' people.

High cholesterol

High blood cholesterol also increases your risk of heart disease. Your blood cholesterol is determined by genetic (inherited) factors, which you cannot change, and lifestyle factors, which you can change.

There are some relatively rare genetic conditions in which particularly high blood cholesterol levels occur. People who have inherited these conditions need a thorough examination by a specialist doctor followed by life-long drug treatment.

In most people, high blood cholesterol is partly determined by their genes, which have 'set' the cholesterol level slightly high, and lifestyle factors which push it up more. Body weight also affects blood cholesterol—in some people, being overweight has a significant effect on the levels, so attaining a reasonable weight can be helpful. The most important dietary factor is fat, in particular, saturated fat. Diets recommended for blood cholesterol lowering are low fat (particularly saturated fat), high carbohydrate, high fibre diets.

The blood also contains triglycerides, another type of fat which may be linked with increased risk of heart disease in some people. Levels of both cholesterol and triglyceride need to be checked as part of an assessment of your risk of heart disease.

High cholesterol foods?

Many people who aim to lower their risk of heart disease focus on avoiding foods that are high in cholesterol. But this is putting the emphasis in the wrong place. Cholesterol itself is concentrated in very few foods (see below) and is not the main cause of our high blood cholesterol levels. In fact, the amount of cholesterol we obtain from food is generally much less than the amount of cholesterol our body makes. Our body can make all the cholesterol we need, but in certain circumstances, our body makes more cholesterol than necessary. This causes the level of cholesterol in our blood to build up and become a problem.

Very few foods are high in cholesterol. Those which are include:

- brains, liver and kidney
- egg yolk
- caviar

A diet high in saturated fat is the biggest contributor to high blood cholesterol. Reducing saturated fat intake can usually improve blood cholesterol levels. Recent work has shown that cholesterol absorption in the gut varies between individuals, thus some individuals are more sensitive to dietary cholesterol than others.

CRP (C-reactive protein)

CRP in the blood is a new and powerful risk factor for heart disease. It is a measure of chronic low grade inflammation, indicative of the damaging effect of high glucose levels and other factors on the blood vessel walls. In women, it predicts future risk of heart disease better than cholesterol levels. Together, CRP and your cholesterol level are a new way for doctors to sort out those at greater risk.

Studies from Harvard have shown that the level of CRP is higher in women ingesting high GI/high glycaemic load diets. That's one more good reason to choose low GI!

Healthy ranges for:	
Cholesterol	< 5.2 mmol/L
Triglycerides	1.0–2.3 mmol/L
HDL cholesterol	1.0–2.5 mmol/L
Total cholesterol/HDL ratio*	< 4.5
Fasting glucose	3.5–6.0 mmol/L
Non-fasting glucose	< 11.1
Glycated haemoglobin	3.5–6.0%
Insulin	< 80 pmol/L
*(no disadvantage to HDL > 2.5)	

OBESITY AND HEART DISEASE

Overweight and obese people are more likely to have high blood pressure and to have diabetes. They are also at increased risk of developing heart disease. Some of that increased risk is due to the high blood pressure, and the tendency to diabetes, but there is a separate 'independent' effect of the obesity.

Two in three British men are
overweight or obese.
Half of British women are
overweight or obese.

When increased fatness develops it can be distributed evenly all over the body or it may occur centrally—in and around the abdomen (tummy)—a 'pot belly'. This latter form of obesity is strongly associated with heart disease. In fact, you can have a pot belly and still be normal weight. But that extra fat around the middle is playing havoc with your metabolism. Every effort should be made to achieve and maintain a reasonable body weight —especially if your extra weight is 'middle-age spread'

How's your shape?

Fat around the middle part of our body (abdominal fat) increases our risk of heart disease, high blood pressure and diabetes. In contrast, fat on the lower part of the body, such as hips and thighs, doesn't carry the same health risk. Your body shape can be described according to your distribution of body fat as either an 'apple' or a 'pear' shape.

Apple shape
larger waist, smaller hips

Pear shape
smaller waist, larger hips

There are significant health benefits in reducing your waist measurement, particularly if you have an 'apple' shape.

You can easily tell if you are an 'apple' or a 'pear' by placing a tape measure around your waist and then your hips and seeing which is smaller. Ideally the waist is smaller than the hips. If it isn't, you're an apple!

Specifically, the waist measurement for people 19 years and over should be:

- less than 102 cm (40 inches) for men;
- less than 88 cm (35 inches) for women;

If you are overweight, or consider yourself overweight, chances are that you have looked at countless books, brochures and magazines offering a solution to losing weight. New diets or miracle weight loss solutions seem to appear weekly. They are clearly good for selling magazines, but for the majority of people who are overweight the 'diets' don't work—if they did, there wouldn't be so many!

At best—while you stick to it—a 'diet' will reduce your kilojoule/calorie intake. At its worst, a 'diet' will change your body composition for the fatter. This is because many diets employ the technique of drastically reducing your carbohydrate intake to bring about quick weight loss. Once you return to your former way of eating, your body contains a little less muscle mass. With each repetition of a diet you lose more muscle.

Not all foods are equal. When it comes to losing weight, it is not necessarily a matter of reducing how much you eat. Research has shown that the type of food you give your body determines what it is going to burn and what it is going to store as body fat. It has also been revealed that certain foods are more satisfying to the appetite than others.

This is where the GI plays a leading role. Low GI foods have two essential advantages for people trying to lose weight:

1. They fill you up and keep you satisfied for longer.

2. They help you burn more body fat and less muscle.

The International Diabetes Federation has published a new set of criteria for defining the metabolic syndrome to make it easier for doctors to identify people who have the condition (April 2005). For people of European origin, the waist circumference thresholds have been reduced to 94 cm (37 inches) for men and 80 cm (31.5 inches) for women, plus any two of the following four factors:

• raised blood triglyceride (> 1.7 mmol/l)*

- reduced blood hdl cholesterol (< 0.9 mmol/l for men, < 1.1 mmol/l for women)*
- raised blood pressure (systolic = 130 mm hg or diastolic = 85 mm hg)*
- raised fasting plasma glucose (= 5.6 mmol/l) or previously diagnosed type 2 diabetes

For people from South Asia and China the waist circumference thresholds are 90 cm (35.5 inches) for men and 80 cm (31.5 inches) for women; while for people from Japan the thresholds are 85 cm (33.5 inches) for men and 90 cm (35.5 inches) for women. For more information go to: http://www.idf.org/home/

*or receiving treatment for this condition

What's wrong with a low carbohydrate diet?

Although low carb diets may help people lose weight, there are serious doubts about their long term safety. They are high in saturated fat—a risk factor for heart disease and cancer. They are often low in fruit and vegetables and therefore protective micronutrients. And in people with compromised kidney function, the need to filter more nitrogen can lead to kidney failure.

One reason for their popularity is that initial loss is rapid. Within the first few days, the scales will be reading

2 to 3 kilograms (4 to 6½ lbs) lower—the trouble is that some of that weight loss isn't body fat, but muscle mass and water.

People who have followed low carbohydrate diets for any length of time observe that the rate of weight loss plateaus off and they begin to feel rather tired and lethargic. That's not surprising because the availability of glucose fuel to muscle is reduced. Strenuous exercise requires both fat and carbohydrate in the fuel mix. So, in the long term, these low carbohydrate diets may discourage people from the physical exercise patterns that will help them keep their weight under control.

Our advice is that the best diet for weight control is one you can stick to for life—one that includes your favourite foods and which accommodates your cultural and ethnic heritage. Choosing low GI foods will not only promote weight control, it will reduce postprandial glycemia, increase satiety, provide bulk and a rich supply of micronutrients.

Low GI diets are the happy compromise between a low fat diet on one hand and a low carb diet on the other.

Eating to lose weight with low GI foods is easier because you don't have to go hungry, you get to eat your favourite foods, and what you end up with is true fat release.

EXERCISE—WE CAN'T LIVE WITHOUT IT!

These days it is increasingly easy to overeat. Refined foods, convenience foods and fast foods frequently lack fibre and conceal fat so that before we feel full, we have overdosed on calories.

It is even easier not to exercise. With intake exceeding output on a regular basis, the result for too many of us is a couch potato lifestyle and subsequent weight gain.

Why exercise keeps you moving

The effect of exercise doesn't stop when you stop moving. People who exercise have higher metabolic rates and their bodies burn more calories per minute even when they are asleep!

How exercise helps

Regular physical activity can reduce our blood glucose levels, lower our risk of heart and blood vessel disease, lower high blood pressure, increase stamina, reduce stress and help us relax. It is meant for us all.

- Exercise speeds up our metabolic rate. By increasing our calorie expenditure, exercise helps to balance our sometimes excessive kilojoule/calorie intake from food and helps us control our weight.
- Exercise makes our muscles better at using fat as a source of fuel. By improving the way insulin works, exercise increases the amount of fat we burn.

A low GI diet has the same effect. Low GI foods reduce the amount of insulin we need, which makes fat easier to burn and harder to store. Since body fat is what you want to get rid of when you lose weight, exercise in combination with a low GI diet makes a lot of sense!

Remember that reduction in body weight takes time. Even after you've made changes in your exercise habits your weight may not be any different, or change very much, on the scales (this is particularly true in women whose bodies tend to gain muscle and lose fat at the same time). So don't weigh yourself obsessively—use a tape measure around the waist instead.

So what can you do?

We need to adapt our lifestyle to our more calorie-laden diet and fewer physical demands. It's important to catch bursts of physical activity whenever we can to increase our energy output.

Your increased movement may be planned, for example, walking 20 to 30 minutes 6 to 7 days a week. Home-based walking programmes like this seem to be one of the best strategies for increasing physical output. Team up with a friend.

Besides planned activity you simply need to move around more in your day. Some suggestions:

- Never use a lift or an escalator if you can help it!
- Walk gently on a treadmill while you watch the news or talk on the telephone.
- Hide the remote control.
- Walk to the corner shops.
- Dance with your kids.
- Park a hundred metres or more from work.
- Take the dog for a walk.
- Have one car-free day every week.
- Limit TV viewing to less than 2 hours a day.
- Buy a step-counter and walk 10 000 steps a day.

Personal trainers can help you to stick to an exercise programme, if you are willing to pay for the privilege of being regularly motivated by someone with appropriate skills.

Whatever it takes for you, do it. Regard movement as an opportunity to improve your mental and physical well-being and not an inconvenience.

Cardiovascular fitness

Cardiovascular fitness is improved by regular strenuous exercise so that the blood supply to the heart may be 'improved'. Specifically, cardiovascular fitness is improved by exercise which is aerobic. This means activity that makes your heart beat faster so your pulse increases and you breathe more deeply.

Current thinking has it that we need to accumulate at least 30 minutes each day of this level of exertion to maintain cardiovascular fitness. Exercise is also important in maintaining body weight and has effects on metabolism and some factors related to blood clotting.

Getting regular exercise is clearly important. So don't just think about it, just do it!

How to make your exercise successful

Some key factors to make exercise successful include:

* seeing a benefit for yourself (e.g. your clothes fit);
* enjoying what you do;
* feeling that you can do it fairly well;
* fitting in with your daily life; and
* being inexpensive and accessible.

THE GI AND THE METABOLIC SYNDROME

Surveys show that 1 in 2 British adults over 25 years of age has at least two features of what is seen to be a silent disease: the metabolic syndrome, or insulin resistance syndrome. This syndrome (sometimes called syndrome X) is a collection of metabolic abnormalities that 'silently' increase your risk of heart attack. The list of features is getting longer and longer, and the number of diseases linked to insulin resistance is growing.

The metabolic syndrome is set to be the disease of the early 21st century.
One in two adults are likely to suffer from the debilitating effects of this condition.

Insulin resistance

In this condition the body is insensitive, or 'partially deaf', to insulin. The organs and tissues that ought to respond to even a small rise in insulin remain unresponsive. The body tries harder by secreting more insulin to achieve the same effect, just as you might raise your voice or shout for a hard-of-hearing person. Thus high insulin levels are part and parcel of insulin resistance. Tests on patients with the metabolic syndrome show that insulin resistance is very common.

You probably have insulin resistance if you have two or more of the following:

• high blood pressure
• low HDL-cholesterol levels
• high waist circumference
• high uric acid levels in blood
• 'pre-diabetes'
• fasting glucose greater than 6 millimoles per litre
• post-glucose load greater than 7.8 millimoles per litre
• high triglycerides

Chances are your total cholesterol levels are within the normal range, giving you and your doctor a false impression of your coronary health.

You might also be normal weight (or overweight) but your waist circumference is high (more than 88 cm (35 inches) in women, more than 102 cm (40 inches) in men), indicating excessive fat around the abdomen.

But the red flag is that your blood glucose and insulin levels after a glucose load, or after eating, remain high. Resistance to the action of insulin is thought to underlie and unite all the features of this cluster of metabolic abnormalities.

One of the questions that's often asked is why insulin resistance is so common. We know that both genes and environment play a role. People of Asian or Indian origins appear to be more insulin resistant than those of European extraction, even when they are still young and lean.

But regardless of ethnic background, insulin resistance develops as we age. This has been attributed not to age per se, but to the fact that as we get older, we gain excessive fat around our middle, we become less physically active and we lose some of our muscle mass. It's also likely that diet plays a role—high fat diets have been associated with insulin resistance; high carbohydrate diets with improving insulin sensitivity.

Insulin resistance as we age results in the metabolic syndrome and gradually lays the foundations of a heart attack and other diseases (stroke, polycystic ovarian syndrome, fatty liver, acne, cognitive impairment).

How can the GI help?

Can a low GI diet help? In a recent study, patients with serious disease of the coronary arteries were given either low or high GI diets before surgery for coronary bypass grafts. They were given blood tests before their diets and just before surgery, and at surgery small pieces of fat tissue were removed for testing.

The tests on the fat showed that the low GI diets made the tissues of these 'insulin insensitive' patients more sensitive—in fact they were back in the same range as normal 'control' patients after just a few weeks on the low GI diet.

If people with serious heart disease can be improved would the same happen with younger people? In another study, young women in their thirties were divided into those who did and those who did not have a family history of heart disease. They themselves had not yet developed the condition. They had blood tests followed by low or high GI diets for four weeks, after which they had more blood tests, and then when they had surgery (for conditions unrelated to heart disease) pieces of fat were again removed and tested for insulin sensitivity. The young women with a family history of heart disease were insensitive to insulin originally (those without the family history of heart disease were normal) but after four weeks on the low GI diet their insulin sensitivity was back within the normal range.

In both studies the diets were designed to try to ensure that all the other variables (total energy, total carbohydrates) were not different, so that the change in insulin sensitivity was likely to have been due to the low GI diet rather than any other factor. For more detailed information on how low GI carbs help you lose weight consult *The Low GI Diet*.

**Research strongly suggests
low GI diets improve the sensitivity
of the body to insulin.**

Polycystic ovarian syndrome (PCOS)

Polycystic ovarian syndrome occurs in women when multiple cysts form on the ovaries during the menstrual cycle and interfere with normal ovulation. Acne and facial hair are part of the problem, as well as being overweight, especially around the middle. PCOS is often diagnosed when women have irregular periods or find it difficult to fall pregnant.

It is now known that insulin resistance is often severe in women with PCOS and that any means of improving insulin sensitivity (drugs, weight loss) will improve outcomes. Some doctors have found that low GI diets are particularly useful for women with PCOS but, at present, there is little research to back this up. However, since low GI diets will help reduce weight and have been shown to improve insulin sensitivity in individuals at risk of coronary heart disease, it makes a lot of sense to try the low GI approach. For more detailed information on how you can improve insulin sensitivity and manage the symptoms of PCOS consult *The Low GI Guide to Managing PCOS*.

Low GI diets

Work on these exciting findings continues but what is known so far strongly suggests that low GI diets not only improve blood glucose in people with and without diabetes, but also the sensitivity of the body to insulin. It will take many years of further research to show that this simple dietary change will definitely slow the progress of atherosclerosis. In the meantime it is clear that risk factors for heart disease are improved by eating a low GI diet.

Low GI diets are consistent with the other required dietary changes needed for prevention of heart disease: they are bulky; filling; high in micronutrients, anti-oxidants and good fats; and help weight control.

Food *without* Exercise = Fat

HOW DOES YOUR DIET RATE?

Reducing the GI of your diet will reduce insulin levels and increase the potential for fat burning. You can achieve an effective reduction in the GI by substituting at least one high GI carbohydrate choice at each meal with a low GI food. It's the carbohydrate foods that you eat the most of which have the greatest impact—so check your intake in the following quiz.

You don't have to avoid all
high GI foods to eat a low GI diet.
Try and eat one low GI food per meal.

What type of carbohydrate did you eat yesterday?

1. Recall the carbohydrate-rich foods that you ate yesterday. Remember to think of snacks as well as the main meals!
2. Tick the check boxes below for the types of foods you ate.

High GI	Low GI

Starchy foods

- ☐ Potato, including baked, mashed, steamed, boiled and chips
- ☐ Rice (American long-grain, instant rice, jasmine)

Starchy foods

- ☐ Sweetcorn
- ☐ Baked beans
- ☐ Sweet potato
- ☐ Chickpeas
- ☐ Kidney beans, lentils
- ☐ Pasta
- ☐ Noodles
- ☐ Basmati rice

Bread Products

- ☐ White bread
- ☐ Wholemeal bread
- ☐ Crumpets
- ☐ Croissants
- ☐ Scones
- ☐ Bagels
- ☐ French bread

Bread Products

- ☐ Wholegrain bread
- ☐ Fruit loaf, raisin toast
- ☐ Sourdough bread

THE LOW GI GUIDE

High GI	Low GI
Cereals	**Cereals**
☐ Cornflakes™	☐ Special K™
☐ Rice Pops™	☐ Porridge
☐ Coco Pops™	☐ Muesli
☐ Puffed Wheat	☐ All-Bran™
☐ Weet-a-Bix™	☐ Frosties™
Biscuits	**Biscuits**
☐ Water crackers	☐ Rich Tea™
☐ Rice cakes	☐ Oatmeal
☐ Digestive biscuits	
☐ Shortbread	
Snacks	**Snacks**
☐ Dates	☐ Dried apricots
☐ Glucose	☐ Prunes
☐ Sweets	☐ Nuts
☐ Pretzels	☐ Yoghurt
☐ Muesli bar	☐ Milk
	☐ Ice-cream
Fruit	**Fruit**
☐ Watermelon	☐ Apples
☐ Dates	☐ Oranges
	☐ Bananas
	☐ Grapes
	☐ Kiwi fruit
	☐ Peaches, plums, apricots

3. Now add up the number of ticks in each column of foods. The foods in the left column have a high GI. If most of your ticks are in this column, you are eating a high GI diet. Consider altering some of your choices to include more of the foods from the column on the right.

Is your diet too high in fat?

Use this fat counter to tally up how much fat your diet contains. Circle all the foods that you could eat in a day, look at the serving size listed and multiply the grams of fat up or down to match your serving size. For example, with milk, if you estimate you might consume 2 cups (500 ml) of regular milk in a day, this supplies you with 20 grams of fat.

Food	Fat content (grams)	How much did you eat?
Dairy Foods		
Milk (250 ml) 1 cup		
regular	10	_____
fat-reduced (less than 1% fat)	1	_____
skimmed	0	_____
Yoghurt, 200 gram tub		
Regular	6	_____
Low fat	0	_____
Ice-cream, 2 scoops (100 ml/50 grams)		
regular, vanilla	5	_____
reduced fat, vanilla	3	_____

Food	Fat content (grams)	How much did you eat?
Cheese		
regular traditional cheese, 20 gram slice	7	_____
reduced-fat block cheese, 30 gram slice	5	_____
low fat slices (per slice)	2	_____
cottage, 2 tablespoons	2	_____
ricotta, 2 tablespoons	2	_____
Cream/sour cream, 1 tablespoon		
regular	7	_____
fat-reduced	5	_____
Fats and oils		
Butter/margarine, 1 teaspoon	4	_____
Oil, any type, 1 tablespoon (20 ml)	20	_____
Cooking spray, per spray	1	_____
Mayonnaise, 1 tablespoon	6	_____
Salad dressing, 1 tablespoon	5	_____
Meat		
Beef		
steak, 1 medium (160 grams), fat trimmed	5	_____
minced beef patty (170 grams), cooked, drained	21	_____
sausage, 1 thick, grilled (80 grams)	13	_____
topside roast, 2 slices, lean only (80 grams)	5	_____
Lamb		
chump chop, grilled/BBQ, 2, fat trimmed	10	_____
leg, roast meat, lean only, 2 slices (60 grams)	6	_____
loin chop, grilled/BBQ, 2, lean only	6	_____

Food	Fat content (grams)	How much did you eat?
Pork		
bacon, I rasher, grilled	6	_____
ham, I slice, leg, lean	I	_____
butterfly steak, fat trimmed	3	_____
leg, roast meat, 3 slices (80 grams) lean only	6	_____
large chop, fat trimmed	9	_____
Chicken		
breast, skinless, 150 grams	8	_____
drumstick, skinless	8	_____
thigh, skinless	12	_____
½ barbecue chicken (including skin)	17	_____
Fish		
grilled fish, I average fillet	3	_____
salmon, 50 grams	5	_____
fish fingers, 4 grilled	10	_____
fish fillets, 2, crumbed, oven baked		
regular	20	_____
light	16	_____
Snack foods		
Chocolate (50 gram bar)	25	_____
Potato crisps (50 gram bag)	15	_____
Corn chips (50 gram bag)	14	_____
Peanuts, ½ cup (70 grams)	36	_____
French fries, regular serve	20	_____
Pizza, 2 slices, medium pizza	18	_____
Pie/sausage roll	17	_____

Total

How did you rate?

Less than 40 grams — Excellent. 30 to 40 grams of fat per day is an average range recommended for those trying to lose weight.

41–60 grams — Good. A fat intake in this range is recommended for most adult men and women.

61–80 grams — Acceptable, if you are very active, i.e. doing hard physical work (labouring) or athletic training. It is too much if you are trying to lose weight.

More than 80 grams — You're possibly eating too much fat, unless of course you are Superman or Superwoman!

EATING THE LOW GI WAY

Low GI diets are easy to teach and easy to learn. The basic technique is to swap high GI carbohydrates in your diet with low GI foods. This could mean eating muesli at breakfast instead of wheat flakes, low GI bread instead of normal white or wholemeal bread, or a sparkling apple juice in place of a soft drink, for example. We've identified some key points that are crucial in putting the GI into practice. Remember:

- *The GI only relates to carbohydrate-rich foods*

The foods we eat contain three main nutrients—protein, carbohydrate and fat. Some foods, such as meat, are high in protein, while bread is high in carbohydrate and butter is high in fat. It is necessary for us to consume a variety of foods (in varying proportions) to provide all three nutrients, but the GI applies only to high carbohydrate foods. It is impossible for us to measure a GI value for foods which contain negligible carbohydrate. These foods include meats, fish, chicken, eggs, cheese, nuts, oils, cream, butter and most vegetables. There are other nutritional aspects which you could consider in choosing these foods. For example, the amount and type of fats they contain.

- *The GI is not intended to be used in isolation*

The GI of a food does not make it good or bad for us. High GI foods like potatoes and bread still make valuable nutritional contributions to our diet. And low GI foods like pastry that are high in saturated fat are no better for us because of their low GI. The nutritional benefits of different foods are many and varied, and it is advisable for you to base your food choices on the overall nutritional content of a food, particularly considering the saturated fat, salt and fibre in addition to GI.

- *There is no need to eat only low GI foods*

While most of us will benefit from eating carbohydrate with a low GI at each meal, this doesn't mean consuming it to the point of exclusion of all other carbohydrate. When we eat a combination of low and high GI carbohydrate foods, like baked beans on toast, fruit and sandwiches, lentils and rice, potatoes and corn, the final GI of the meal is moderate/medium. The high GI of foods like potatoes is moderated by including a low GI carbohydrate at the same meal. For example, if your main meal contains Desiree potatoes with a GI of 91, then choose a low GI dessert like low fat yoghurt with a GI of 33. Let's assume that half the carbohydrate comes from the potato and half from the yoghurt. The GI for the meal then becomes $(50\% \times 91) + (50\% \times 33) = 62$.

- *Consider both the GI of the food and the amount of carbohydrate it contains, i.e. the glycaemic load*

For a small number of foods, the normal serving size contains so little carbohydrate that the GI of that carbohydrate is unimportant. This is the case for fruits like watermelon (GI of 76) and for vegetables like parsnips (GI of 97) and pumpkin (GI of 75) which provide about 6 grams of carbohydrate per serving. Small amounts of jam (strawberry jam has a GI of 51) or honey (with an average GI of 55) also have little glycaemic impact. You can calculate the glycaemic load by multiplying the GI by the amount of carbohydrate per serve and then dividing by 100. We have included the glycaemic load of foods in the tables at the end of the book.

High GI food + Low GI food =
moderate/medium GI meal

Glycaemic load =
(GI x carbohydrate per serve) ÷ 100

As with the kilojoule/calorie content of foods, the GI value is not precise and gives only an estimate. What GI values give you is a guide to lowering the GI of your day. A simple change can make a big difference. Look at the type of carbohydrate foods you eat and identify those which you eat the most (these generally have the greatest glycaemic load). Consider the high carbohydrate foods you consume at each meal and replace at least one with a low GI food (e.g. replace potatoes with sweet potatoes). This will result in a significant reduction in the overall GI of your diet. Look at the following table for substitution suggestions.

Substituting low GI for high GI foods

High GI Food	Low GI Alternative
Bread, wholemeal or white	Bread containing a lot of 'grainy bits' such as multigrain or granary loaves
Processed breakfast cereal	Unrefined cereal such as rolled oats or muesli or a low GI processed cereal like All-Bran™
Plain biscuits and crackers	Biscuits made with dried fruit and whole grains such as oats
Cakes and muffins	Make them with fruit, oats, whole grain
Potato	Substitute with new potatoes, sweet potatoes, sweetcorn and use more pasta and legumes
Rice	Try Basmati rice, or pearl barley, quinoa or noodles

Making the change

Some people change their diet easily, but for the majority of us, change of any kind is difficult. Changing our diet is seldom just a matter of giving up certain foods. A healthy diet contains a wide variety of foods but we need to eat them in appropriate proportions. If you are considering changes to your diet, keep these four guidelines in mind:

1. Aim to make changes gradually.

2. Attempt the easiest changes first.

3. Break big goals into a number of smaller, more achievable goals.

4. Accept lapses in your habits.

If you feel like you need some extra help, seek some professional assistance from a dietitian.

5 little tips that make a big difference

- Think of carbohydrate foods as the number one priority in your meals.
- Change a staple in your diet, like bread, to a low GI type to make a big difference to the GI of your day.
- Get in touch with your true appetite and use it to guide the amount of food you eat. Low fat, high fibre, low GI foods fill you up best.
- Try to eat at least two low GI meals each day.
- Mix high GI foods with low GI foods in your meals— the combination will give an overall intermediate GI.

HOW TO FIND A DIETITIAN

For specific information about your own kilojoule and exact carbohydrate needs, you should consult a registered dietitian (RD). For a list of registered dietitians, visit the website www.bda.uk.com. Alternatively, send a self-addressed envelope to the British Dietetic Association (BDA), in order to receive a list of registered dietitians. The list will have the RD names, locations and telephone numbers. The address of the BDA is: 5th Floor Charles House, 148/9 Great Charles Street, Queens Way, Birmingham, B3 3HT.

In addition, the following website provides specific information about dietitians specialising in the GI: www.diagnosemefirst.com.

Make sure that the person you choose has the letters RD after his or her name.

TEN STEPS TO A HEALTHY HEART DIET

1. Eat more wholegrain breads and cereals.

2. Use beans, peas and lentils more often.

3. Eat lots of fruit and vegetables.

4. Include oily fish at least twice a week
   e.g. salmon, sardines.

5. Minimise saturated fats.

6. Reduce your use of salt.

7. Moderate your alcohol intake.

8. Include unsalted nuts in your diet in moderation.

9. Use low fat dairy products.

10. Allow yourself a treat a day.

1. Eat more wholegrains

Wholegrains represent the earliest form in which humans consumed cereals. Eaten boiled or roughly pounded to a flour, mixed with water and roasted, they were a form of slow-release carbohydrate with a low GI. They were also filling and sustaining. The advent of high speed roller mills in the Industrial Revolution led to the development of the fine, white flour that is used today. Because the outer seed coat has been removed, the starch in today's flour is readily digested and has a high GI.

We can still get the benefit of wholegrains in our diet today with foods like:

- barley—e.g. pearl barley in soup;
- whole wheat or cracked wheat e.g. bulghur in tabbouli;
- oats and rolled oats for breakfast; and
- wholegrain breads (the ones with chewy grains and seeds).

If you are making your own bread, GI lowering ingredients to add include linseeds, rolled oats, cornmeal, oat bran, barley meal and kibbled wheat.

2. Use more dried peas, beans and lentils

Dried peas, beans and lentils are collectively known as legumes. They are an excellent food, being:

- rich in low GI carbohydrate
- low in fat
- high in fibre
- low cost

Because they are high in protein, legumes are an ideal substitute for meat. Introduce them to your family gradually by incorporating them in meals with meat e.g. as chilli con carne, a filling for tacos or burritos, and then try some of the delicious vegetarian dishes that can be made using legumes. You could also try:

- 3-bean mix with a salad
- a can of kidney beans in a bolognese sauce
- hommous dip or spread
- pea and ham soup
- potato bake with beans and lean bacon

The special benefits of soya

Foods based on soya beans also have a beneficial role in our defence against heart disease. There are two components of soya beans with the potential to reduce coronary heart disease risk: soya protein and anti-oxidant substances called 'isoflavones'.

Soya foods:

- improve blood fats—lowering the bad (LDL) cholesterol;
- increase the good (HDL) cholesterol;
- reduce the accumulation of cholesterol in blood vessels by decreasing LDL oxidation and thereby inflammation;
- decrease the tendency to form blood clots or thromboses; and
- have other health promoting effects on blood vessels.

Studies suggest that 1–2 servings of soya protein-rich food each day may be sufficient to provide long term health benefit. Just one cup of soya drink constitutes a serving and can be used as a nutritionally balanced replacement for dairy milk providing it is fortified with calcium. Try:

- soya drink on your breakfast cereal
- a soya banana smoothie
- a soya yoghurt for a snack

3. Eat lots of fruit and vegetables

Plant foods are rich sources of naturally occurring chemicals believed to be involved in disease prevention. Increased consumption of fruit and vegetables is associated with a lower incidence of diseases such as cancer, cardiovascular disease and other age-related diseases.

At least 5 servings a day of fruit and vegetables is recommended. These foods are an essential source of vitamin C but also rich in anti-oxidants and fibre.

Get into a fruit and vegetable habit:

- Don't sit down to a main meal without some vegetables in it.
- Take an apple and a banana to work.
- Make a habit of eating some fruit at home when you relax in the evening.
- Order a side salad with your meal.
- Buy a new vegetable to try each week.
- Consider fresh, canned, dried and juiced fruit as sources of fruit for your diet.
- Chop fresh pineapple or melon into large chunks and keep it on hand in the refrigerator.
- Prepare a fruit platter for the household to share after a meal.

4. Include oily fish at least twice a week

Oily fish are the best source of long chain omega-3 fatty acids. These types of fats are scarcely found in other foods and offer valuable benefits in reducing blood clotting and inflammatory reactions. They can help in the prevention and treatment of heart disease, high blood pressure and rheumatoid arthritis. They are also beneficial in infant brain and eye development.

Fresh fish that are highest in omega-3 fats include:

- atlantic salmon
- herring
- silver perch
- mackerel—fresh and smoked
- sardines
- kippers
- mullet
- sturgeon
- salmon—fresh and smoked

Canned fish can also provide substantial amounts of omega-3 fat. Good sources are:

- mackerel
- salmon
- sardines

Smoked salmon and mackerel and oysters are also a rich source.

Aim to include fish in your diet at least twice a week e.g. a main meal of fresh fish NOT cooked in saturated fat, plus at least one sandwich-sized serving of, say, canned salmon.

A WORD ABOUT FISH AND MERCURY

While there are many benefits of eating fish, if you are pregnant you do need to be careful about the types of fish you eat. Some fish contain high levels of mercury which can be harmful to your baby.

FSA (Food Standards Agency United Kingdom) recently revised their guidelines on mercury in fish. They advise that pregnant women, women planning pregnancy and young children can continue to consume a variety of fish as part of a healthy diet but should limit their consumption of certain species. Shark (flake), marlin and swordfish should be consumed no more than once per fortnight with no other fish to be consumed during that fortnight. For orange roughy (also sold as sea perch) and catfish, their advice is to consume no more than one serve per week, with no other fish being consumed during that week. Most other varieties of fish caught and sold in the UK contain low levels of mercury and can be eaten without concern.

For more information on the subject consult the website www.food.gov.uk.

5. Reduce saturated fats

Approximately 40 per cent of fats in the British diet are saturated fats. This type of fat is believed to be a major cause of high cholesterol levels in our population. The main sources are:

- full cream dairy foods, especially milk, cheese, cream
- ice-cream products
- fat spreads, especially butter, cream cheese and cheese spreads
- take-away foods like deep fried foods, chips, pizza
- snack foods like potato crisps, biscuits, cakes
- fatty meat like sausage and salami

Make every effort to reduce your intake of saturated fats by eating less of the foods listed previously. Substitute with unsaturated fats where possible, for example:

Instead of:	Substitute:
butter	monounsaturated spread e.g. olive oil spread
dripping/lard	polyunsaturated or monounsaturated oil
regular milk	low fat or skimmed milk
fatty meat	smaller amounts of leaner cuts
regular ice-cream	one of the many low fat varieties on the market
regular cheese	eat it occasionally; try low fat and reduced fat alternatives

What fat is that?

The fat in our food is a combination of different types of fatty acids. Depending on which fatty acids predominate, we identify the fat as either saturated, monounsaturated or polyunsaturated.

Saturated	Monounsaturated	Polyunsaturated
Butter	Olive oil margarine	Polyunsaturated margarines
Solid cooking fats	Rapeseed oil	Sunflower oil
	Olive oil	Safflower oil
Palm oil	Peanut oil	Soyabean oil
Coconut oil	Avocado	Walnuts
	Peanuts	Hazelnuts
	Almonds	Brazil nuts
Cocoa butter	Peanut butter	Sunflower seeds

6. Minimise use of salt

It has been estimated that 75 per cent of the salt we eat is not from that which we voluntarily add, but from salt already existing in foods. Bread and butter/margarine, for example, contribute much of the salt we eat. Low salt breads take some time to adjust your tastebuds to, but low salt margarines are easy to find on the supermarket shelves and are not noticeably different in taste.

Foods that are high in salt include:

- canned, bottled and packet soups, sauces and meal and gravy bases, stock cubes
- ham, bacon, sausages and other delicatessen meats
- pizza, meat pies, sausage rolls, fried chicken and other take-away foods
- pickles, chutneys, olives
- snack foods like potato crisps

7. Consume alcohol in moderation

There is no doubt that large quantities of alcohol should be avoided, but several studies have suggested that a moderate alcohol intake can exert a protective effect against heart disease in some people.

People who drink 1–2 standard drinks per day, but not necessarily every day, show a reduced risk of heart disease, with the effect being greatest amongst those with other risk factors for heart disease. The effect of alcohol may be mediated through an increase in the level of 'good' HDL cholesterol. Anti-oxidant substances in red wine which reduce the oxidation of 'bad' LDL cholesterol are also thought to be involved.

It is important to note the finding that 3 or more drinks per day actually increases the risk of death!

A standard drink in the UK contains about 8 g of alcohol— the amount found in half a pint of ordinary strength beer or one small glass (125 ml) of wine, or a single measure of spirits.

8. Include nuts in your diet

Nuts are a food that many people enjoy but few people eat regularly—a situation that needs to change! Large prospective studies in recent years have found a strong link between higher consumption of nuts and reduced risk of heart disease. Nuts contain a very favourable mix of fatty acids which have a positive effect on blood fat levels.

Nuts are also a good source of other nutrients thought to protect against heart disease including vitamin E, folate, copper and magnesium.

Because they are so nutrient and energy dense, nuts need only be eaten in small quantities.

While sitting down to a bowl of nuts may not be such a good idea if you are trying to lose weight, consuming small amounts of nuts regularly is quite healthy. Try:

• chopped almonds or pecans in a muesli
• a snack of nuts and dried fruit
• toasted cashews to finish a stir-fry
• a handful of pine nuts scattered over a salad

9. Use low fat dairy products

Dairy foods supply about 70 per cent of our calcium needs and contribute low GI carbohydrate to our diet. Low fat flavoured milks, custards, yoghurts, ice-creams and mousse make great-tasting snacks and desserts.

Men and pre-menopausal women should aim to consume 700 mg of calcium each day. After menopause, optimal intakes for women are up to 1500 mg a day. This requires at least three ½ pint (250 ml) servings of low fat milk products daily.

Low fat milk supplies as much (and usually more) calcium than full cream milk so is entirely suitable for those wanting to increase their calcium intake.

- ½ pint (250 ml) of low fat milk contains about 415 mg of calcium and only 0.5 g of fat.
- ½ pint (250 ml) of regular milk contains about 295 mg of calcium and 9.7 g of fat.

Full cream milk is recommended for children under 5 years of age because young children have a greater reliance on the calories provided by fat.

10. Allow yourself a treat

Food is meant to be enjoyed!

Allow yourself to indulge in a little of whatever takes your fancy but check with yourself that it is what you really feel like. Indulgences are meant to be enjoyed:

- your favourite cheese and crackers
- a hot dog at the football
- bacon and egg on Sundays
- a take-away on Friday night
- a slice of cake at a celebration
- chocolate biscuits with a friend

The message for heart disease prevention is low fat (low saturated fat), high carbohydrate, high fibre and low GI most of the time!

YOUR LOW GI
STOCKLIST

Nothing affects our day-to-day food choices as much as what we have in the cupboard. Use these ideas as the basis of your shopping list.

Breads
All types of bread are suitable but the lowest GI choices are:

> Burgen™ varieties such as Soya and Linseed
> Vogels™ varieties

Spreads
If you wish to use a fat spread on your bread choose a margarine labelled 'polyunsaturated' or 'monounsaturated' (and preferably salt reduced).

Breakfast cereals

All-Bran™—try all varieties (Kellogg's)

Special K™ (Kellogg's)

Natural muesli or low fat toasted muesli

Rolled oats (porridge) and oat bran

Fruits

Lowest GI fresh fruit choices include:

Apples	Plums	Grapefruit
Bananas	Peaches	Berries (all)
Pears	Oranges	Grapes

Dried fruits—sultanas, dried apricots, fruit medley, raisins, prunes etc.

Canned peaches, pears, apples are a useful standby.

Fruit juices are also suitable but shouldn't be drunk to excess —generally only ½–1 pint (250–500 ml) per day.

Rice & grains

Basmati rice

Pasta—fresh and dried

Noodles—fresh and dried

Pearl barley

Quinoa

Bulghur

Legumes

Dried lentils, chick peas, cannellini beans

A variety of canned legumes (kidney beans, mixed beans, baked beans)

Vegetables

All vegetables are good for you—fresh, frozen and canned.
Raw salad vegetables are available partially prepared to make
a quick addition to the meal. Canned vegetables—tomatoes,
asparagus, peas, corn, beetroot, mushrooms and crisp, canned
mixed vegetables are always handy to boost the vegetable
content of a meal. Other convenient vegetable products are:

> tomato paste
> tomato purée and bottled tomato pasta sauces
> frozen vegetables

Meats

Any meat trimmed of all visible fat
Low fat minced meat
Skinless chicken or turkey
Lean bacon
Lean cold meats—ham, corned beef, pastrami, turkey or
  chicken breast

Fish

All fresh fish is recommended
Canned fish such as salmon, mackerel, tuna, herrings, sardines
Smoked fish, like smoked cod
Frozen fish products that have used polyunsaturated or
  monounsaturated oils in their preparation (check labels
  carefully!)

Seafood

Most seafood is suitable to include regularly but avoid if
  battered or crumbed or in a creamy sauce.

Dairy foods

Milk—fat-reduced and skimmed

Yoghurt—low fat, fruit and natural

UHT skimmed milk or skimmed milk powder—easy to use in cooking

Canned evaporated skimmed milk

Low fat ice-cream

Cottage cheese, low fat ricotta

Low fat traditional and processed cheese (check the label for those that are less than 10 per cent fat.)

Flavourings, sauces & dressings

Spices—curry powder, cumin, turmeric, mustard etc.

Herbs—oregano, basil, thyme etc.

Bottled minced ginger, chilli and garlic

Sauces e.g. Worcestershire, soya, chilli, oyster, BBQ, hoisin

Stock base or powders

Low oil salad dressings

A WEEK OF LOW GI EATING

This week of menus shows you how to achieve a healthy heart diet with a low GI. You can use the menus for ideas for your own meal choices or follow them closely to try out the low GI diet.

We have included a couple of between-meal snacks in most of the menus as they can be part of a normal healthy diet.

Each menu is designed to be:

- **low in fat, especially saturated fat**
  We've kept the total amount of fat down to provide less than 30 per cent of total calories, according to current recommendations. Saturated fat content is less than 20 grams per day.

- **low in kilojoules/calories**
  These menus provide a total daily kilojoule/calorie intake of between 5800 and 7000 kJ (1400–1700 cal) which is a minimum amount for most people. Be guided by your appetite to adjust quantities to suit yourself.

- **high in carbohydrate with a low GI**
  The carbohydrate content of these menus provides at least 50 per cent of total kilojoule/calorie intake. This means an intake of at least 200 grams of carbohydrate each day. The emphasis is on low GI carbohydrate choices.

Generally, beverages are included only where they make a significant nutrient or kilojoule/calorie contribution. Supplement the menus with a range of fluids such as water, tea, coffee, herbal tea, cereal coffee, mineral water and soda with lemon or lime juice.

Recipe ideas for dishes marked with an asterisk are given on pages 94–96.

Note: 1 calorie = energy needed to raise temperature of 1 litre of water by 1 degree Celsius.
1 calorie = 4.2 kilojoules

Making a meal of it

Here are the three simple steps to putting together a balanced low GI meal.

Step 1: **Carbohydrate** is an essential, although sometimes forgotten part of a balanced meal. What do you feel like? Potato, rice, pasta, noodles? Include at least one low GI carb per meal.

Step 2: Include some **protein** at each meal. It lowers the glycaemic load and low glycaemic-load meals produce smaller increases in blood sugar than do high glycaemic-load meals.

Step 3: If anything, **fruit and vegetables** really ought to have the highest priority, but a meal based solely on fruit and low carbohydrate vegetables won't be sustaining for long.

This plate model is adaptable to serves of any size.

* As long you keep food to the proportions shown here, the meal will be a balanced one.
* And as long as the types of food you choose fit within the guidelines for healthy eating, then you should have a good diet overall.

1 Carbohydrate
2 Protein
3 Vegetables

Monday Menu

Total Energy:	6300 kJ/1500 Cal
Saturated Fat:	10 g
Carbohydrate:	230 g
Fibre:	44 g

Breakfast:
A bowl of All-Bran™ with a sliced banana
and low fat milk
Slice of grain toast with unsaturated
margarine

Morning snack
A couple of oatmeal biscuits

Lunch:
Two slices of grainy bread filled with
tuna, lettuce and mayonnaise. Follow
with a serving of canned fruit

Dinner:
A large bowl of steaming, thick minestrone
soup served with crusty Italian bread and a
salad with vinaigrette dressing

Night snack
One scoop of low fat, low GI ice-cream
with fresh fruit salad

Tuesday Menu

Total Energy: ....6400 kJ/1524 Cal
Saturated Fat: ....10 g
Carbohydrate: ....230 g
Fibre: ....33 g

Breakfast: Top a couple of slices of raisin loaf with low fat ricotta cheese and a finely sliced pear. Finish with a hot chocolate made with low fat milk

Lunch: A baked bean toasted sandwich (spray the sandwich maker with cooking spray) and a cup of fresh pineapple chunks

Afternoon snack   A low fat apple muffin

Dinner: Barbecued Beef Kebabs* with Quick Rice Combo* and a side salad or steamed vegetables

Night snack   Lemon sorbet

* See recipes on pages 95–96

Wednesday Menu

Total Energy: ....6000 kJ/1429 Cal
Saturated Fat: ....12 g
Carbohydrate: ....200 g
Fibre: ....30 g

Breakfast:
A bowl of porridge with a tablespoon of sultanas and low fat milk, with a glass of orange juice

Lunch:
Two slices of grain bread spread with avocado, topped with beetroot, grated carrot and lettuce. A piece of fresh fruit and water

Afternoon snack
A tub of low fat yoghurt

Dinner:
Quick Vegetarian Pizza* and a side salad

Night snack
A small handful (30 g) of almonds and a glass of sparkling apple juice

* See recipe on page 94

Thursday Menu

Total Energy: ....7000 kJ/1667 Cal
Saturated Fat: ....12 g
Carbohydrate: ....230 g
Fibre: ....40 g

Breakfast: Toast 2 slices of grain bread and top with a smear of avocado, sliced tomato and black pepper. Add a piece of fresh fruit and a drink

Lunch: Try a bowl of lentil and vegetable soup with Lebanese flat bread, or pita bread

Afternoon snack An orange

Dinner: Salmon Cakes* served with a medley of baby corn, mangetouts, sliced carrots and spring onions. Drizzle with sweet chilli sauce if desired

Night snack Low fat ice-cream in a cone

* See recipe on page 95

Friday Menu

Total Energy:	5800 kJ/1381 Cal
Saturated Fat:	15 g
Carbohydrate:	180 g
Fibre:	32 g

Breakfast: Top a couple of slices of grain toast with baked beans and a poached egg. Add a small glass of grapefruit juice or fresh grapefruit

Lunch: Two slices of sourdough rye bread, smear of light cream cheese, sliced smoked salmon and a side salad

Afternoon snack A slice of raisin toast with a scrape of margarine

Dinner: Easy Creamy Pasta* with tomato topping and side salad

Night snack A tub of frozen yoghurt

* See recipe on page 94

Saturday Menu

Total Energy:	7000 kJ/1667 Cal
Saturated Fat:	8 g
Carbohydrate:	230 gl
Fibre:	44 g

Breakfast: A bowl of Special K® with low fat milk, low fat berry yoghurt and a handful of strawberries

Lunch: A pita bread filled with felafel, hommous, tomato, lettuce, tabbouli and chilli sauce

Afternoon snack   Small bunch of grapes

Dinner: Moroccan Lamb and Spicy Rice* and steamed vegetables

Night snack   2 fresh plums

* See recipe on page 95

Sunday Menu

Total Energy:	6600 kJ/1571 Cal
Saturated Fat:	12 g
Carbohydrate:	175 g
Fibre:	30 g

Breakfast: A bowl of fresh fruit salad topped with 100 g (3½ oz) low fat fruit yoghurt. Add a reduced fat apple and sultana muffin

Lunch: Whip up an omelette and serve it with a couple of slices of grain bread. Combine 1 whole egg with 2 beaten egg whites. Cook lightly in an omelette pan and top with diced tomato, spring onions and a sprinkle of grated reduced fat cheese. Finish under the grill

Afternoon snack A banana

Dinner: Pan-cook or barbecue a fish cutlet drizzled with a little olive oil, lemon juice, salt and pepper. Serve with canned new potatoes and steamed seasonal vegetables

Night snack A glass of fruit juice and a small scoop of cashews

QUICK MEAL IDEAS

These recipe ideas are used in the previous menu plans. The quantities are only a rough guide and can be adjusted to taste.

Easy Creamy Pasta

Put 250 g (10 oz) of broad fettuccine noodles on to boil. Combine 50 g (2 oz) of fresh ricotta, 50 g (2 oz) of low fat natural yoghurt, 50 g (2 oz) of grated parmesan and 3 teaspoons of margarine. Stir this mixture through the drained pasta, adding some sautéed onion and garlic for extra flavour if desired. A quick topping idea is bottled pasta sauce.

Serves 4.

Quick Vegetarian Pizza

Sauté a diced onion, a clove of crushed garlic and strips of green pepper. Add 4 thinly sliced mushrooms and basil and oregano to taste and cook 5 minutes. Stir in a small can of red kidney beans.

Sprinkle a pizza base with 100 g (4 oz) of grated reduced fat mozzarella or pizza cheese. Spoon the bean mixture over. Pour over about 100 g (4 oz) of bottled tomato puree and top with another 100 g (4 oz) of cheese. Bake 10–15 minutes in a hot oven.

Serves 4.

Salmon Cakes

Combine 200 g (8 oz) canned salmon with half a finely diced onion, 100 g (4 oz) of mashed potato, 2 teaspoons chopped parsley and 1 egg. Shape into patties and cook in a pan sprayed with cooking spray.

Serves 2.

Moroccan Lamb & Spicy Rice

Coat about 120 g (4 oz) of trim lamb (e.g. lamb fillet) with a commercial Moroccan spice blend and pan-fry in a little oil. Remove to a plate and keep warm. In the same pan, sauté a finely sliced onion until golden, collecting the spice remaining in the pan. Add 200 g (8 oz) of cooked Basmati rice and 50 g (4 oz) of cooked baby peas. Stir over heat to combine and heat through. Serve topped with the lamb cut into strips and freshly steamed vegetables.

Serves 1.

Quick Rice Combo

Stir fry 2 rashers of trimmed, diced bacon, 1 small red pepper, diced, 2 chopped shallots, 200 g (8 oz) of frozen corn/peas and 100 g (8 oz) of bean sprouts. Add 400 g of cooked Basmati rice, drizzle with soya sauce and serve.

Serves 2.

Barbecued Beef Kebabs

Marinate approximately 500 g (18 oz) of diced beef (e.g. rump, fillet) in 125 ml (4 fl oz) red wine, 1 tbspn vinegar, 1 tbspn olive oil, 1 tspn Worcestershire sauce, 2 tbspns tomato sauce, crushed garlic and black pepper. Thread onto skewers alternately with button mushrooms, diced pepper and diced onion. Grill or barbecue and serve with Quick Rice Combo (page 95).

Serves 4.

Vegetables

Pile your plate high with leafy green and salad vegetables and eat your way to long-term health and vitality.

Think of vegetables as 'free' foods that are full of fibre, essential nutrients and protective anti-oxidants that will fill you up without adding extra calories. And most are so low in carbohydrate that they will have no measurable effect on your blood glucose levels.

Leafy green and salad vegetables, for example, have so little carbohydrate that we can't test their GI. Even in generous serving sizes, they will have no effect on your blood glucose levels.

LET'S TALK GLYCAEMIC LOAD

When we eat a meal containing carbohydrate, our blood glucose rises and falls. The extent to which it rises and remains high is critically important to health and depends on two things: the *amount* of a carbohydrate in the meal and the *nature* (GI) of that carbohydrate. Both are equally important determinants of changes in blood glucose levels.

Researchers at Harvard University have come up with a way of combining and describing these two factors with the term 'glycaemic load'. Glycaemic load is the product of the GI and carbohydrate per serve of food. You'll find it listed in the tables at the back of this book.

Glycaemic load is calculated simply by multiplying the GI of a food by the amount of carbohydrate per serving and dividing by 100.

Glycaemic load = (GI × carbohydrate per serving) ÷ 100

For example, an apple has a GI of 40 and contains 15 grams of carbohydrate per serve. Its glycaemic load is (40 × 15) ÷ 100 = 6.

A potato has a GI of 90 and 20 grams of carbohydrate per serve. It has a glycaemic load of (90 × 20) ÷ 100 = 18.

The glycaemic load is greatest for those foods which provide the most carbohydrate, particularly those we tend to eat in large quantities. Compare the glycaemic load of the following foods to see how the serving size as well as the GI are significant in determining the glycaemic response:

Rice—1 serve (150 g) of boiled Calrose rice contains 43 g carbohydrate and has a GI of 83. The glycaemic load is (43 × 83) ÷ 100 = 36.

Spaghetti—1 serve (150 g) of cooked spaghetti contains 48 g carbohydrate and has a GI of 44. The glycaemic load is (48 × 44) ÷ 100 = 21.

Some nutritionists have argued that the glycaemic load is an improvement on the GI because it provides an estimate of both quantity and quality of carbohydrate (the GI gives us just quality) in a diet. In large scale studies from Harvard University, however, the risk of disease was predicted by both the GI of the overall diet as well as the glycaemic load. The use of the glycaemic load strengthened the relationship, suggesting that the more frequent the consumption of high carbohydrate, high GI foods, the more adverse the health outcome.

Don't make the mistake of using GL alone. If you do, you might find yourself eating a diet with very little carbohydrate but a lot of fat, especially saturated fat, and excessive amounts of protein. Use the glycaemic index to compare foods of similar nature (e.g. bread with bread) and use the glycaemic load when you note a high GI but low carbohydrate content per serve (e.g. watermelon).

So what should you do?

- Use the GI to compare foods of a similar nature (breads with breads); the low GI varieties will have the lower GI values.
- Use the GL when comparing foods with a high GI but low carbohydrate content per serving.

A TO Z
GI & GL TABLES

These A to Z tables will help you put those low GI food choices into your shopping trolley and onto your plate. To make an absolutely fair comparison, all foods are tested following an internationally standardised method. Gram for gram of carbohydrates, the higher the GI, the higher the blood glucose levels after consumption.

> A **low** GI value is 55 or less
> A **moderate/medium** GI value is 56 to 69 inclusive
> A **high** GI value is 70 or more

To give you the full picture of the glycaemic impact of foods, the tables in this book also include the GL (glycaemic load) of average sized portions of the food on your plate. Glycaemic load is the product of GI and the amount of carbohydrate in a serving of food. This means that you can choose foods with either a low GI and/or a low GL.

A **low** GL value is 10 or less
A **moderate/medium** GL value is 11 to 19 inclusive
A **high** GL value is 20 or more

Use the GI tables to:
- identify the best carbohydrate choices
- find the GI of your favourite foods
- compare carb-rich foods within a category (two types of bread or breakfast cereal for example)
- improve your diet by finding a low GI substitute for high GI foods
- put together a low GI meal
- help you calculate the GL of a meal or serving if it is more or less than our specified nominal portion size

Use the GL tables to:
- find foods with a high GI but low carbohydrate content per serving

Remember, the GL values listed in these tables are for the specified nominal portion size. If you eat more (or less) you will need to calculate another GL value.

We have also included some foods that contain very little carbohydrate or none at all in these tables because so many people ask us for their GI. Many vegetables such as avocado and broccoli, and protein rich foods such as eggs, cheese, chicken and tuna are among the low or no carbohydrate category. Most alcoholic beverages are also low in carbohydrate.

* indicates that this food contains little or no carbohydrate

In addition, not all low GI foods are a good choice; some are too high in saturated fat and sodium for everyday eating.

■ indicates that this food is high in saturated fat. As we have mentioned before, the GI should not be used in isolation, but the overall nutritional value of the food needs to be considered.

If you can't find the GI value for a food you regularly eat in these tables, check out our website (www. glycaemicindex.com). We maintain an international database of published GI values that have been tested by a reliable laboratory. Alternatively, contact the manufacturer and encourage them to have the food tested by an accredited laboratory. In the meantime, choose a similar food from the tables as a substitute.

Look for the GI on the foods you buy

A GI symbol on the packet tells you that a food has been glycaemic index tested. Unfortunately, not all claims are reliable.

The GI Symbol Programme

This symbol on foods is your guarantee that the product meets the GI Symbol Programme's strict nutritional criteria. Whether high, medium or low GI, you can be assured that these foods are * healthier choices within their food group and will make a nutritious contribution to your diet.

The GI Symbol Programme is an international programme that was established by the University of Sydney, Diabetes Australia and the Juvenile Diabetes Research Foundation—organisations whose expertise in GI is recognised around the world. The logo is a trademark of the University of Sydney in Australia and in other countries including the UK. A food product carrying this logo is nutritious and has been tested for its GI in an accredited laboratory. For more information, visit www.gisymbol.com

Some UK supermarket chains are progressively testing and labelling their foods. But at the time of going to press, the GI values have not been released for publication. We will include these foods in our

---

* ©® and ™ University of Sydney in Australia and other countries. All rights reserved.

comprehensive tables as soon as they become available and we have had an opportunity to evaluate them.

- **Sainsbury's** are launching GI labelling progressively across a range of products that meet strict nutritional criteria and backing this with a comprehensive guide to GI on their website (www.sainsburys.co.uk). The products have been tested by Hammersmith Hospital Food Research Company.

- **Tesco** have had a number of foods glycaemic index tested by Oxford Brookes University and these foods are labelled low or medium GI (www.tesco.com).

Note: The GI values in this book are correct at the time of publication. However, the formulation of commercial foods can change and the GI may change as well.

FOOD	GI	NOMINAL SERVE SIZE	AVAILABLE CARB PER SERVE	GL PER SERVE	
Alfalfa sprouts	*	6 g	0	0	A
All-Bran®, breakfast cereal, Kellogg's®	34	30 g	15	4	
Angel food cake, plain	67 ■	50 g	29	19	
Apple, dried	29	60 g	34	10	
Apple, fresh	38	120 g	15	6	
Apple juice, Granny Smith, pure	44	200 ml	24	10	
Apple juice, no added sugar	40	250 ml	28	11	
Apple muffin, home-made	46 ■	60 g	29	13	
Apricots, canned in light syrup	64	120 g	19	12	
Apricots, dried	30	60 g	28	9	
Apricots, fresh	57	168 g	13	7	
Arborio, risotto rice, white, boiled	69	150 g	43	29	
Artichokes, globe, fresh or canned in brine	*	80 g	0	0	
Arugula	*	30 g	0	0	
Asparagus	*	100 g	0	0	
Aubergine	*	100 g	0	0	
Avocado	*	120 g	0	0	
Bacon	*	50 g	0	0	B
Bagel, white	72	70 g	35	25	
Baked beans, canned in tomato sauce	49	150 g	17	8	
Banana cake, home-made	51 ■	80 g	38	18	
Banana, raw	52	120 g	26	13	
Banana smoothie, low fat	30	250 ml	22	7	
Barley, pearled, boiled	25	150 g	32	8	
Basmati rice, white, boiled	58	150 g	38	22	
Bean curd, tofu, plain, unsweetened	*	100 g	0	0	
Bean sprouts, raw	*	14 g	0	0	
Bean thread noodles, dried, boiled	33	180 g	45	12	
BEANS, PEAS & LEGUMES					
Kidney beans, dark red, canned, drained	43	150 g	25	7	
Kidney beans, red, canned, drained	36	150 g	17	9	
Kidney beans, red, dried, boiled	28	150 g	25	7	
Beef	*	120 g	0	0	
Beetroot, canned	64	80 g	7	5	

* little or no carbs ■ high in saturated fat

FOOD	GI	NOMINAL SERVE SIZE	AVAILABLE CARB PER SERVE	GL PER SERVE
Biscuits, digestive, plain	59 ■	25 g	16	10
Biscuits, Rich Tea®	55 ■	25 g	19	10
Biscuits, shortbread, plain	64 ■	25 g	16	10
Biscuits, wafer, vanilla, plain	77 ■	25 g	18	14
Black bean soup, canned	64	250 ml	27	17
Black beans, boiled	30	150 g	25	5
Black rye bread	76	30 g	13	10
Black-eyed beans, soaked, boiled	42	150 g	29	12
Blueberry muffin, commercially made	59 ■	57 g	29	17
Bok choy	*	100 g	0	0
Borlotti beans, canned, drained	41	75 g	12	5
Bran Flakes™, breakfast cereal, Kellogg's®*	74	30 g	18	13
Bran muffin, commercially made	60 ■	57 g	24	15
Brawn	* ■	75 g	0	0
BREADS				
Bun, hamburger, white	61	30 g	15	9
Dark rye bread	86	30 g	14	12
Fruit loaf, thick sliced	47	30 g	15	7
Light rye bread	68	30 g	14	10
Melba toast, plain	70	30 g	23	16
Multigrain sandwich bread	65	30 g	28	18
Organic stoneground wholemeal sourdough bread	59	32 g	12	7
Pita bread, white	57	30 g	17	10
Pumpernickel bread	50	30 g	10	5
Roll (bread), white	73	30 g	16	12
Sourdough rye bread	48	30 g	12	6
Sourdough wheat bread	54	30 g	14	8
Soya and Linseed, Bürgen®	55	70 g	24	13
White bread, regular, sliced	71	30 g	14	10
BREAKFAST CEREALS				
All-Bran®, Kellogg's®	34	30 g	15	5
Bran Flakes, Kellogg's®	74	30 g	18	13
Coco Pops®, Kellogg's®	77	30 g	26	20

* little or no carbs ■ high in saturated fat

FOOD	GI	NOMINAL SERVE SIZE	AVAILABLE CARB PER SERVE	GL PER SERVE
BREAKFAST CEREALS				
Corn Flakes®, Kellogg's®	77	30 g	25	20
Crunchy Nut Corn Flakes Bar, Kellogg's®	72	30 g	26	19
Crunchy Nut Corn Flakes, breakfast cereal, Kellogg's®	72	30 g	24	17
Frosties®, Kellogg's®	55	30 g	26	15
Oat bran, raw, unprocessed	55	10 g	5	3
Oats, rolled, raw	59	50 g	31	18
Porridge, instant, made with water	82	30 g	26	17
Porridge, regular, made from oats with water	58	250 g	21	11
Puffed Wheat	80	30 g	21	17
Rice Krispies®, Kellogg's®	82	30 g	26	22
Semolina, cooked	55	150 g	11	6
Shredded Wheat	75	30 g	20	15
Special K®, regular, Kellogg's®	56	30 g	21	11
Sultana Bran™, Kellogg's®	73	30 g	19	14
Broad beans	79	80 g	11	9
Broccoli	*	60 g	0	0
Brussels sprouts	*	100 g	0	0
Buckwheat, boiled	54	150 g	30	16
Buckwheat, puffed	65	14 g	12	8
Bulghur, cracked wheat, ready to eat	48	150 g	26	12
Bun, hamburger, white	61	30 g	15	9
Butter beans, canned, drained	36	75 g	12	4
Butter beans, dried, boiled	31	150 g	20	6
Cabbage	*	70 g	0	0
Cake, chocolate, made from packet mix with icing	38 ■	111 g	52	20
Cake, cupcake, strawberry-iced	73 ■	38 g	26	19
Cake, pound, plain	54 ■	50 g	23	12
Cake, sponge, plain, unfilled	46 ■	63 g	36	17
Calamari rings, squid, not battered or crumbed	*	70 g	0	0
Cannellini beans	31	85 g	12	4

C

* little or no carbs ■ high in saturated fat

FOOD	GI	NOMINAL SERVE SIZE	AVAILABLE CARB PER SERVE	GL PER SERVE
Cantaloupe	67	120 g	6	4
Carrot juice, freshly made	43	250 ml	23	10
Carrots, peeled, boiled	41	80 g	5	2
Cashew nuts, salted	22	30 g	9	2
Cauliflower	*	60 g	0	0
Celery	*	40 g	0	0
CEREAL GRAINS				
Rye, grain	34	50 g	38	13
Cheese	*■	120 g	0	0
Cheese tortellini, cooked	50■	180 g	21	10
Cherries, dark, raw	63	120 g	12	3
Chicken	*	110 g	0	0
Chicken nuggets, frozen, reheated in microwave 5 mins	46■	100 g	16	7
Chickpeas, canned in brine	40	150 g	22	9
Chickpeas, dried, boiled	28	150 g	24	7
Chillies, fresh or dried	*	20 g	0	0
Chives, fresh	*	4 g	0	0
Chocolate cake, made from packet mix with icing	38■	110 g	52	20
Chocolate, dark, plain	41■	30 g	19	8
Chocolate, milk, plain, Cadbury's®	49■	30 g	17	8
Chocolate, white, plain, Nestlé®	44■	50 g	29	13
Coca-Cola®, soft drink	53	250 ml	26	14
Coco Pops®, breakfast cereal, Kellogg's®	77	30 g	26	20
Condensed milk, sweetened, full fat	61■	50 ml	28	17
Consommé, clear, chicken or vegetable	*	205 g	2	0
Corn, sweet, on the cob, boiled	48	80 g	16	8
Corn, sweet, whole kernel, canned, drained	46	80 g	14	7
Cornflakes, breakfast cereal, Kellogg's®	77	30 g	25	20
Cornmeal (polenta), boiled	68	150 g	13	9
Courgette	*	100 g	0	0
Couscous, boiled 5 mins	65	150 g	33	21

* little or no carbs ■ high in saturated fat

FOOD	GI	NOMINAL SERVE SIZE	AVAILABLE CARB PER SERVE	GL PER SERVE
Cranberries, dried, sweetened	64	40 g	29	19
Cranberry Juice Cocktail, Ocean Spray	52	250 ml	31	16
Croissant, plain	67 ■	57 g	26	17
Crumpet, white	69	50 g	19	13
Crunchy Nut Corn Flakes Bar, Kellogg's®	72	30 g	26	19
Crunchy Nut Corn Flakes Bar, Kellogg's®	72	30 g	26	19
Cucumber	Q	45 g	0	0
Cupcake, strawberry-iced	73 ■	38 g	26	19
Custard apple, fresh, flesh only	54	120 g	19	10
Custard, home-made from milk, wheat starch and sugar	43 ■	100 ml	17	7
Custard, vanilla, reduced fat	37	100 ml	15	6
Dark rye bread	86	30 g	14	12
Dates, Arabic, dried, vacuum-packed	39	55 g	41	16
Dates, dried	103	60 g	40	42
Desiree potato, peeled, boiled 35 mins	101	150 g	17	17
Diet jelly, made from crystals with water	*	125 g	0	0
Diet soft drinks	*	250 ml	0	0
Digestive biscuits, plain	59 ■	25 g	16	10
Dried apple	29	60 g	34	10
Duck	* ■	140 g	0	0
Eggs	* ■	120 g	0	0
Endive	*	30 g	0	0
Fanta®, orange soft drink	68	250 ml	34	23
Fat-free yoghurts, various flavours	40	200 g	31	12
Fennel	*	90 g	0	0
Fettuccine, egg, cooked	40	180 g	46	18
Figs, dried, tenderised	61	60 g	26	16
Fish	*	120 g	0	0
Fish fingers	38 ■	100 g	19	7
Four bean mix, canned, drained	37	75 g	12	5
French fries, frozen, reheated in microwave	75 ■	150 g	29	22
Frosties®, breakfast cereal, Kellogg's®	55	30 g	26	15
Fructose, pure	19	10 g	10	2

D

E

F

* little or no carbs ■ high in saturated fat

FOOD	GI	NOMINAL SERVE SIZE	AVAILABLE CARB PER SERVE	GL PER SERVE
Fruit loaf, thick sliced	54	30 g	15	8
G Garlic	*	5 g	0	0
Ginger	*	10 g	0	0
Glucose tablets	100	10 g	10	10
Glutinous rice, white, cooked in rice cooker	98	150 g	32	31
Gnocchi, cooked	68	180 g	48	33
Golden syrup	63	20 g	17	11
Granny Smith apple juice, unsweetened	44	200 ml	24	10
Grapefruit, fresh	25	120 g	11	3
Grapefruit juice, unsweetened	48	250 ml	22	9
Grapes, fresh	53	120 g	18	8
Green beans	*	70 g	0	0
Green pea soup, canned	66	250 ml	41	27
H Ham, leg or shoulder	*■	24 g	0	0
Hamburger bun, white	61	30 g	15	9
Haricot beans, cooked, canned	38	150 g	31	12
Haricot beans, dried, boiled	33	150 g	31	12
Heinz® Baked Beans in tomato sauce, canned	49	150 g	17	8
Herbs, fresh or dried	*	2 g	0	0
Hommous, regular	6	30 g	5	1
Honey and Oat Bran bread, Vogel's	49	40 g	13	7
Honey, pure floral	35	25 g	18	6
Honey, various (averaged)	55	25 g	18	10
I Ice-cream, vanilla, full fat	38■	50 g	9	3
Instant mashed potato	85	150 g	20	17
Instant noodles, 99% fat free	67	75 g	51	34
Instant noodles, regular	54■	180 g	23	10
Instant rice, white, cooked 6 mins	87	150 g	42	36
Isostar® sports drink	70	250 ml	18	13
J Jasmine rice, white, long-grain, cooked in rice cooker	109	150 g	42	46
Jelly beans	78	30 g	28	22
Jelly, diet, made from crystals with water	*	125 g	0	0

* little or no carbs ■ high in saturated fat

FOOD	GI	NOMINAL SERVE SIZE	AVAILABLE CARB PER SERVE	GL PER SERVE
Kidney beans, dark red, canned, drained	43	150 g	25	7
Kidney beans, red, canned, drained	36	150 g	17	9
Kidney beans, red, dried, boiled	28	150 g	25	7
Kiwi fruit, fresh	53	120 g	12	6
Lamb	*	120 g	0	0
Leeks	*	80 g	0	0
Lemon	*	40 g	0	0
Lentil soup, canned	44	250 ml	21	9
Lentils, green, dried, boiled	30	150 g	17	5
Lentils, red, dried, boiled	26	150 g	18	5
Lettuce	*	50 g	0	0
Licorice, soft	78	60 g	42	33
Light rye bread	68	30 g	14	10
Lima beans, baby, frozen, reheated in microwave	32	150 g	30	10
Lime	*	40 g	0	0
Linguine pasta, thick, durum wheat, boiled	46	180 g	48	22
Linguine pasta, thin, durum wheat, boiled	52	180 g	45	23
Linseed and Soya Loaf, bread	55	70 g	24	13
Liver sausage	*■	30 g	0	0
Low fat soya milk, calcium-fortified	44	250 ml	17	8
Lucozade®, original, sparkling glucose drink	95	250 ml	42	40
Lychees, canned, in syrup, drained	79	120 g	20	16
M&M's®, peanut	33 ■	30 g	17	6
Macaroni, white, plain, boiled	47	180 g	48	23
Mango, fresh	51	120 g	17	8
Maple syrup, pure, Canadian	54	24 g	18	10
Mars Bar®, regular	62 ■	60 g	40	25
Marshmallows, plain, pink and white	62	25 g	20	12
Melba toast, plain	70	30 g	23	16
Milk, semi-skimmed, low fat (1.4%)	32	250 ml	12	4
Milk, skimmed, low fat (0.1%)	32	250 ml	12	4

K

L

M

* little or no carbs ■ high in saturated fat

FOOD	GI	NOMINAL SERVE SIZE	AVAILABLE CARB PER SERVE	GL PER SERVE
Milk, soya, calcium-enriched	36	250 ml	18	6
Milk, soya, calcium-enriched	36	250 ml	18	6
Milky Bar®, plain white chocolate, Nestlé®	44 ■	50 g	29	13
Minestrone soup, traditional, canned	39	250 g	18	7
Muesli bar, chewy, with choc chips or fruit	54 ■	31 g	21	12
Muesli bar, crunchy, with dried fruit	61	30 g	21	13
Muffins, apple, home-made	46 ■	60 g	29	13
Muffins, blueberry, commercially made	59 ■	57 g	29	17
Muffins, bran, commercially made	60 ■	57 g	24	15
Multigrain sandwich bread	65 ■	30 g	28	18
Mung bean noodles (bean thread), dried, boiled	33	180 g	45	18
Mung beans	39	150 g	17	5
Mushrooms	*	35 g	0	0
New potato, canned, microwaved 3 mins	65	150 g	18	12
New potato, unpeeled and boiled 20 mins	78	150 g	21	13
Noodles, 2 minute regular, Maggi	54	75 g	51	34
Noodles, 2 minute (99% fat free), Maggi	71	75 g	51	34
Nutella®, hazelnut spread	33	20 g	12	4
Nuts, peanuts, roasted, salted	14	50 g	6	1
Nuts, pecan, raw	10	50 g	3	1
Oat bran, unprocessed	55	10 g	5	3
Oatcakes	57 ■	25 g	15	8
Oats, rolled, raw	59	50 g	31	18
Okra	*	80 g	0	0
Onions, raw, peeled	*	30 g	0	0
Orange, fresh	42	120 g	11	5
Orange juice, unsweetened	50	250 ml	18	9
Organic stoneground wholemeal sourdough bread	59	32 g	12	7
Oysters, natural, plain	*	85 g	0	0
Parsnips	97	80 g	12	12

* little or no carbs ■ high in saturated fat

FOOD	GI	NOMINAL SERVE SIZE	AVAILABLE CARB PER SERVE	GL PER SERVE
PASTA				
Cheese tortellini, cooked	50 ■	180 g	21	10
Fettuccine, egg, cooked	40	180 g	46	18
Gnocchi, cooked	68	180 g	48	33
Linguine, thick, durum wheat, boiled	46	180 g	48	22
Linguine, thin, durum wheat, boiled	52	180 g	45	23
Macaroni, white, plain, boiled	47	180 g	48	23
Ravioli, meat-filled, durum wheat flour, boiled	39 ■	180 g	38	15
Rice pasta, brown, boiled	92	180 g	38	35
Spaghetti, white, durum wheat, boiled 10–15 mins	44	180 g	48	21
Spaghetti, wholemeal, boiled	42	180 g	42	16
Spirali, white, durum wheat, boiled	43	180 g	44	19
Vermicelli, white, durum wheat, boiled	35	180 g	44	16
Paw paw, fresh	56	120 g	8	5
Peach, fresh	42	120 g	11	5
Peaches, canned, in heavy syrup	58	120 g	15	9
Peaches, canned, in light syrup	57	120 g	18	9
Peaches, canned, in natural juice	45	120 g	11	4
Peanuts, roasted, salted	14	50 g	6	1
Pear, fresh	38	120 g	11	4
Pear halves, canned, in natural juice	44	120 g	13	5
Pear halves, canned, in reduced-sugar syrup	25	120 g	14	4
Peas, dried, boiled	22	150 g	9	2
Peas, green, frozen, boiled	48	80 g	7	3
Pecan nuts, raw	10	50 g	3	1
Pineapple, fresh	59	120 g	10	6
Pineapple juice, unsweetened	46	250 ml	34	16
Pita bread, white	57	30 g	17	10
Pizza, Super Supreme, pan, Pizza Hut	36 ■	100 g	24	9
Pizza, Super Supreme, thin and crispy, Pizza Hut *	30 ■	100 g	22	7
Plum, raw	39	120 g	12	5

* little or no carbs ■ high in saturated fat

FOOD	GI	NOMINAL SERVE SIZE	AVAILABLE CARB PER SERVE	GL PER SERVE
Polenta, boiled	68	150 g	13	9
Polos®	70	30 g	30	21
Pop-Tarts™, chocotastic	70	50 g	36	25
Popcorn, plain, cooked in microwave	72	20 g	11	8
Pork	*■	120 g	0	0
Porridge, instant, made with water	82	30 g	26	17
Porridge, regular, made from oats with water	58	250 g	21	11
Potato crisps, plain, salted	54■	50 g	18	10
POTATOES				
Desiree, peeled, boiled 35 mins	101	150 g	17	17
French fries, frozen, reheated in microwave	75■	150 g	29	22
Instant mashed potato	85	150 g	20	17
New, canned, microwaved 3 mins	65	150 g	18	12
New, unpeeled, boiled 20 mins	78	150 g	21	13
Sweet potato, baked	46	150 g	25	11
Pound cake, plain	54■	50 g	23	12
Pretzels, oven-baked, traditional wheat flavour	83	30 g	20	16
Prunes, pitted	29	60 g	33	10
Puffed rice cakes, white	82	25 g	21	17
Puffed Wheat, breakfast cereal	80	30 g	21	17
Pumpernickel bread	50	30 g	10	5
Pumpkin	75	80 g	4	3
Quinoa, organic, boiled	53	100 g	17	9
Radishes	*	15 g	0	0
Raisins	64	60 g	44	28
Raspberries	*	65 g	0	0
Ravioli, meat-filled, durum wheat flour, boiled	39■	180 g	38	15
Rhubarb	*	125 g	0	0
Rice cakes, puffed, white	82	25 g	21	17
Rice noodles, dried, boiled	61	176 g	39	24
Rice noodles, fresh, boiled	40	180 g	39	15
Rice pasta, brown, gluten-free, boiled	92	180 g	38	35

Q
R

* little or no carbs ■ high in saturated fat

FOOD	GI	NOMINAL SERVE SIZE	AVAILABLE CARB PER SERVE	GL PER SERVE
Rice vermicelli, dried, boiled	58	180 g	39	22
Risotto rice, Arborio, boiled	69	150 g	43	29
Rockmelon	65	12 g	6	4
Roll (bread), white	73	30 g	16	12
Rye bread, wholemeal	51	40 g	13	7
Rye, grain	34	50 g	38	13
Ryvita® crispbread*	69	25 g	16	11
Salami	*■	120 g	0	0
Salmon, fresh or canned in water or brine	*	150 g	0	0
Sardines	*	60 g	0	0
Sausages, fried	28 ■	100 g	3	1
Scallops, natural, plain	*	160 g	0	0
Scones, plain, made from packet mix	92	25 g	9	8
Semolina, cooked	55	150 g	11	6
Shallots	*	10 g	0	0
Shredded Wheat breakfast cereal	75	30 g	20	15
Skimmed milk, low fat (0.1%)	32	250 ml	12	4
Skittles®	70 ■	50 g	45	32
Sourdough bread, organic, stoneground, wholemeal	59	32 g	12	7
Sourdough rye bread	48	30 g	12	6
Sourdough wheat bread	54	30 g	14	8
Soya and Linseed, Bürgen®	55	70 g	24	13
Soya milk, calcium-enriched	36	250 ml	18	6
Soya milk, low-fat, calcium-fortified	44	250 ml	17	8
Soya yoghurt, Peach and Mango, 2% fat	50	200 g	26	13
Soyabeans, canned	14	150 g	6	1
Soyabeans, dried, boiled	18	150 g	6	1
Spaghetti, gluten-free, rice and split pea, canned in tomato sauce	68	220 g	27	19
Spaghetti, white, durum wheat, boiled 10–15 mins	44	180 g	48	21
Spaghetti, wholemeal, boiled	42	180 g	42	16
Special K®, regular, breakfast cereal, Kellogg's®	56	30 g	21	11

* little or no carbs ■ high in saturated fat

THE LOW GI GUIDE

FOOD	GI	NOMINAL SERVE SIZE	AVAILABLE CARB PER SERVE	GL PER SERVE
Spinach	*	75 g	0	0
Spirali pasta, white, durum wheat, boiled	43	180 g	44	19
Split pea soup, canned	60	250 ml	27	16
Sponge cake, plain, unfilled	46 ■	63 g	36	17
Spring onions	*	15 g	0	0
Squash, yellow	*	70 g	0	0
Squid or calamari, not battered or crumbed	*	70 g	0	0
Steak, any cut	* ■	120 g	0	0
Strawberries, fresh	40	120 g	3	1
Strawberry jam, regular	51	30 g	20	10
Sugar	68	10 g	10	7
Sultana Bran™, breakfast cereal, Kellogg's®	73	30 g	19	14
Sultanas	56	60 g	45	25
Sushi, salmon	48	100 g	36	17
Swede, cooked	72	150 g	10	7
Sweetcorn, on the cob, boiled	48	80 g	16	8
Sweetcorn, whole kernel, canned, drained	46	80 g	14	7
Sweet potato, baked	46	150 g	25	11
Sweetened condensed full fat milk	61 ■	50 g	28	17
Sweetened dried cranberries	64	40 g	29	19
Taco shells, cornmeal-based, baked	68	20 g	12	8
Tofu (bean curd), plain, unsweetened	*	100 g	0	0
Tomato	*	150 g	0	0
Tomato juice, no added sugar	38	250 ml	9	4
Tomato soup, canned	45	250 ml	17	6
Tortellini, cheese, boiled	50 ■	180 g	21	10
Trout, fresh or frozen	*	63 g	0	0
Tuna, fresh or canned in water or brine	*	120 g	0	0
Turkey	* ■	140 g	0	0
Twix® bar	44 ■	60 g	39	17
Vanilla cake made from packet mix with vanilla frosting,	42 ■	111 g	58	24

* little or no carbs ■ high in saturated fat

FOOD	GI	NOMINAL SERVE SIZE	AVAILABLE CARB PER SERVE	GL PER SERVE
Vanilla custard, reduced fat	37	100 g	15	6
Vanilla ice-cream, full fat	38■	50 g	9	3
Veal	*	120 g	0	0
Vermicelli, white, durum wheat, boiled	35	180 g	44	16
Vinegar	*	5 ml	0	0
Vogel's honey and oat bran bread	49	40 g	13	7
Wafer biscuits, vanilla, plain	77■	25 g	18	14
Water crackers, plain	78	25 g	18	14
Watercress	*	8 g	0	0
Watermelon, raw	76	120 g	6	4
Wheat, cracked, bulghur, ready to eat	48	150 g	26	12
White bread, regular, sliced	71	30 g	14	10
Wholemeal rye bread	51	40 g	13	7
Wild rice, boiled	57	164 g	32	18
Yam, peeled, boiled	37	150 g	36	13
Yoghurt, diet, low fat, no added sugar, vanilla or fruit (averaged)	20	200 g	13	3
Yoghurt, Ski™, low fat, with sugar, Strawberry	33	200 g	31	10

W

Y

Note

The GI of the brand-name items listed in the tables has been derived from *in vivo* testing by reliable laboratories in various countries around the world. Because processing procedures may vary from country to country, products manufactured in the UK may or may not have identical values.

* little or no carbs ■ high in saturated fat

Reading sources and references

Jenkins DJA, Wolever TMS, Taylor RH, et al. 'Glycamic index of foods: a physiological basis for carbohydrate exchange.' *American Journal of Clinical Nutrition* 1981;34: 362–6.

Salmeron J, Manson JE, Stampfer MJ, Colditz GA, Wing AL, Willet WC. 'Dietary fiber, glycemic load and risk of non-insulin-dependent diabetes mellitus in women.' *Journal of the American Medical Association* 1997;277: 472–77.

Salmeron J, Ascherio EB, Rimm GA, Colditz D, Spiegelman D, Jenkins DJ, Stampfer MJ, Wing AL, Willet WC. 'Dietary fiber, glycemic load and risk of NIDDM in men.' *Diabetes Care* 1997;20: 545–50.

Liu S, Stampfer MJ, Manson JE, Hu FB, Franz M, Hennekens CH, Willet WC. 'A prospective study of dietary glycaemic load and risk of myocardial infarction in women.' *The Federation of American Societies for Experimental Biology Journal* 1998;124: A260 (abstract#1517).

Frost G, Keogh B, Smith D, Akinsanya K, Leeds AR. 'The effect of low glycaemic carbohydrate on insulin and glucose response in vivo and in vitro in patients with coronary heart disease.' *Metabolism* 1995;45: 669–72.

Frost G, Keogh B, Smith D, Leeds AR. 'Differences in glucose uptake in adipocytes from patients with and without coronary heart disease.' *Diabetic Medicine* 1998;15: 1003–9.

Frost G, Trew G, Margara R, Leeds AR, Dornhorst A. 'Improvement in adipocyte insulin response to a low glycemic index diet in women at risk of cardiovascular disease.' *Metabolism* 1998;47: 1245–51.

Frost G, Leeds AR, Dore CJB, Madieros S, Brading SA, Dornhorst A. 'Glycaemic index as a determinant of serum high density lipoprotein.' *Lancet* 1999; 353: 1045–8.

Brand-Miller JC. Glycemic load and chronic disease. Nutr Rev. 2003 May;61(5 Pt 2):S49-55.

Brand-Miller JC, Colagiuri S. Evolutionary aspects of diet and insulin resistance. World Rev Nutr Diet. 1999;84:74-105.

Brynes AE, Lee JL, Brighton RE, Leeds AR, Dornhorst A, Frost GS. A low glycemic diet significantly improves the 24-h blood glucose profile in people with type 2 diabetes, as assessed using the continuous glucose MiniMed monitor. Diabetes Care. 2003 Feb;26(2):548-9.

Foster-Powell K, Holt SH, Brand-Miller JC. International table of glycemic index and glycemic load values: 2002. Am J Clin Nutr. 2002 Jul;76(1):5-56.

Hu FB, Willett WC. Optimal diets for prevention of coronary heart disease. JAMA. 2002 Nov 27;288(20):2569-78.

Jenkins DJ, Axelsen M, Kendall CW, Augustin LS, Vuksan V, Smith U. Dietary fibre, lente carbohydrates and the insulin-resistant diseases. Br J Nutr. 2000 Mar;83 Suppl 1:S157-63.

Kelly S, Frost G, Whittaker V, Summerbell C. Low glycaemic index diets for coronary heart disease. Cochrane Database Syst Rev. 2004 Oct 18;(4):CD004467.

Leeds AR. Glycemic index and heart disease. Am J Clin Nutr. 2002 Jul;76(1):286S-9S.

Liu S, Willett WC. Dietary glycemic load and atherothrombotic risk. Curr Atheroscler Rep. 2002 Nov;4(6):454-61.

McKeown NM, Meigs JB, Liu S, Saltzman E, Wilson PW, Jacques PF. Carbohydrate nutrition, insulin resistance, and the prevalence of the metabolic syndrome in the Framingham Offspring Cohort. Diabetes Care. 2004 Feb;27(2):538-46.

McMillan-Price J, Brand-Miller J. Dietary approaches to overweight and obesity. Clin Dermatol. 2004 Jul-Aug;22(4):310-4.

Patel VC, Aldridge RD, Leeds A, Dornhorst A, Frost GS. Retrospective analysis of the impact of a low glycaemic index diet on hospital stay following coronary artery bypass grafting: a hypothesis. J Hum Nutr Diet. 2004 Jun;17(3):241-7.

Skurk T, Hauner H. Obesity and impaired fibrinolysis: role of adipose production of plasminogen activator inhibitor-1. Int J Obes Relat Metab Disord. 2004 Nov;28(11):1357-64.

Trayhurn P, Wood IS. Adipokines: inflammation and the pleiotropic role of white adipose tissue. Br J Nutr. 2004 Sep;92(3):347-55.

Wilkin TJ, Voss LD. Metabolic syndrome: maladaptation to a modern world. J R Soc Med. 2004 Nov;97(11):511-20.

Where to go for help and further information

Your doctor

Your local doctor is a good starting point to assess your risk of heart disease and help you minimise and manage your risk.

A dietitian

For nutritional advice we suggest you seek the service of a dietitian who can provide nutritional assessment and guidance on an appropriate diet. The glycaemic index of foods is a part of dietitians' training, so all dietitians should be able to help you in applying the principles in this book, but some dietitians do specialise in certain areas. If you want specific advice on the glycaemic index, check with the dietitian when booking. You can contact a Registered Dietician through your local hospital or GP practice. Check for the letters RD after their name, which indicates that they are a registered dietitian. For a list of dietitians in private practice in your area contact the British Dietetic Association (BDA). (Phone 0121 200 8080; website www.bda.uk.com)

Heart UK

Heart UK is a non-profit organisation specialising in the treatment of the genetic disorder Familial Hyper-cholesterolaemia (FH), which affects around 120 000 people in the UK who, unless correctly diagnosed and treated, are likely to suffer premature heart attacks or strokes in their 30s and 40s. Heart UK's bimonthly magazine and website include information, news and nutrition and lifestyle advice related to the link between high cholesterol and serious heart disease. (Phone 01628 628 638; website www.heartuk.org.uk)

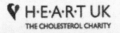

About the authors

Professor Jennie Brand-Miller is Professor of Human Nutrition in the Human Nutrition Unit, School of Molecular and Microbial Biosciences at the University of Sydney, and President of the Nutrition Society of Australia. She has taught postgraduate students of nutrition and dietetics at the University of Sydney for over 25 years and currently leads a team of 12 research scientists. Professor Brand-Miller was recently awarded a Clunies Ross National Science and Technology Medal for her work in championing a new approach to nutrition and the management of blood glucose.

Kaye Foster-Powell is an accredited practising dietitian with extensive experience in diabetes management. A graduate of the University of Sydney (B.Sc., Master of Nutrition & Dietetics) she has conducted research into the glycaemic index of foods and its practical applications over the last 15 years. Currently she is the senior dietitian with Sydney West Diabetes Service and provides consultancy on all aspects of the glycaemic index.

Dr Anthony Leeds is Senior Lecturer in the Department of Nutrition & Dietetics at King's College, London. He graduated in medicine from the Middlesex Hospital Medical School, London, in 1971. He conducts research on carbohydrate and dietary fibre in relation to heart disease, obesity and diabetes and continues part-time medical practice. In 1999 he was elected a Fellow of the Institute of Biology.